LIPOSCULPTURE AND LIPEDEMA SURGERY

A GUIDE FOR THE PATIENT AND PEARLS FOR THE SURGEON

PRAISE FOR LIPOSCULPTURE AND LIPEDEMA SURGERY

"This innovative and scientifically exhaustive solution to the increasing cosmetic, physiologic, and functional damage of lipodystrophy is sine-qua-non with Dr. David Amron. To many, Beverly Hills is to cosmetics is to what Milan, Italy represents to fashion...the epicenter. However, it is a small community of only a few square miles. I have had, over the past 3 decades, the opportunity to observe the incredible legacy constructed by Dr. Amron. To say that David is a pioneer of modern functional and cosmetic dermatological surgery would be a vast understatement. As attested to by his world-wide notoriety; his highly competed-after, top-of-class fellowship; tireless schedule of medical lectures throughout the world; and superhuman surgical schedule, Dr. Amron not only is also relevant today... he leads the direction of the field.

"Personally, and quietly, I have observed an immense loyalty to the science and professional decorum over the years, when the rest of his peers were seduced by Beverly Hills' golden era. This gravitas on his part culminated in the creation of the landmark Roxbury Institute which today is considered a fundamental reference in the science and practice of dermatology and plastic surgery. But David also has a light, personable side, as exemplified by our hit TV series "Dr. 90210," on the E! Entertainment Network. This can be observed in his writing style in this VERY READABLE volume. For the summation of the pioneering mind, excellence in practice, loyalty to the science, and affable style, I recommend this scientific work to all those who aspire to excellence in the field. In fact, failure to carefully study this game-changing work, will compromise one's relevance in the field!"

— Robert Rey, MD. MPP (Harvard '90, '98)
"Dr. 90210" E! Entertainment Network.

"I have admired and respected Dr. Amron's focus and dedication to the field of liposculpture surgery, having worked closely with him for many years. He has earned a worldwide reputation as the pioneer of Lipedema surgery in the United States and has advanced the field of cosmetic and revision liposuction. This book is filled with invaluable information about Dr Amron's unique philosophy and technique, and is a must read for both patients and surgeons."

— Paul Nassif, MD. F.A.C.S.
Board Certified, World-Renowned Facial Plastic and Reconstructive Surgeon, co-host of the E! Entertainment Network reality series Botched.

"It has been my distinct pleasure to be in the operating room and observe Dr. David Amron as he skillfully and methodically orchestrates his surgeries. I am an internationally and nationally certified lymphedema therapist, specializing in the treatment of Lipedema and have over thirty years of experience. I have personally worked with many of Dr. Amron's Lipedema patients postoperatively and have seen the excellent results he has achieved.

"If you want an in-depth understanding of the importance of the lymphatic system and how it relates to Lipedema, this book is a must read. This book has invaluable information for practitioners, patients, and physicians on surgical techniques and postoperative care, based on Dr. Amron's over twenty years of experience.

"I am recommending this book because it clearly gives an understanding of the techniques needed for preparation for Lipedema surgery, during surgery, as well as throughout a patient's care. Dr. Amron's knowledge and understanding of Lipedema and the lymphatic system is evident throughout this book."

— Linda Anne Kahn, CLT-LANA, CDT, NCBTMB.
Certified Lymphedema Therapist.

"Dr. Amron's book is a comprehensive guide that equips patients with the tools and knowledge needed to make an informed choice when considering treatment options and their surgeon. It is a must-read for every Lipedema patient debating liposuction surgery, liposculpture, or nonsurgical body contouring.

"Whether it's complicated revision, Lipedema, or first-time liposuction, this book provides the reader with a deep understanding of who truly qualifies for liposuction surgery and if it is for you."

— Emily Iker, MD.
Director of Lymphedema Center, Santa Monica, CA.

LIPOSCULPTURE AND LIPEDEMA SURGERY

A GUIDE FOR THE PATIENT AND PEARLS FOR THE SURGEON

DAVID M. AMRON, MD.

Published by The Roxbury Institute®.

ISBN: 979-8-218-18787-3

This book is not intended for use as a source of medical advice. The information in this book is intended to provide basic information on Liposuction, Liposculpture, other cosmetic surgery procedures and the subjects discussed. It is not intended to be comprehensive by any means. This book is not intended to diagnose or to treat any medical conditions, or to replace the advice of the reader's physician(s).

The reader should regularly consult a physician in matters related to his or her health, specifically with respect to any symptoms that may require diagnosis or medical attention. For diagnosis or treatment of any medical problems, consult your physician(s).

The author and publisher are not responsible or liable for any damages or negative consequences from any treatment, action, application, or preparation to any person reading or following the information in this book.

While all attempts have been made to verify information provided in this publication, the author and publisher assume no responsibility for errors, omissions, or contrary interpretation of the subject matter herein. Any perceived slights of specific persons or organizations are unintentional. Any trademarks mentioned in this book are listed for reference purposes only and are the property of the respective trademark owners.

I dedicate this book to my parents, Michael and Moselle Amron, who always inspired and guided me to be the best person I can be and to live a good life of purpose and meaning.

I thank my wife, Jessica, and my children Ariel, Benjamin, Abigail, and Asher for their endless love and support.

Finally, I thank my patients for the honor and trust they have placed in me to help them in their journey. They motivate me to excel as a medical professional.

CONTENTS

Preface 1

Introduction 3

Science, Artistry, Engineering, Design, and Execution 4

The History of Liposuction 5

Understanding the Role of Liposuction 7

The "Cosmetic Unit" and the Circumferential Approach 10

Section 1: Cosmetic Liposuction 15

The Three-Dimensional Circumferential Approach 17

Natural Def Lipo 21

The Anesthetic Approach 23

The Process 25

Precision Sculpting: How I Sculpt in the "Safe Plane" 28

The Tools 30

The Treatment Plan 32

Markings and Incision Points 36

Understanding Surface Area and Safe Lidocaine Levels 47

Amount of Fat Removed 50

Gravitationally Prone Areas: Lipoprevention 52

Skin Elasticity and Skin Tightening 54

Cellulite 58

Combining Liposuction with Other Procedures 61

The Preoperative Visit 63

Postoperative Care 65

Results 67

Noninvasive Fat Loss Techniques: Are They Worth It? 71

CONTENTS

Section 2: Revision Liposuction 75

Introduction 77

Emotional Trust of the Patient for Revision Work 79

Complexity of Revision Work 81

Categories of Problems Encountered in Revision Liposuction 82

Strategies and Techniques 91

Strategies to Correct Problems in Revision Liposuction Surgery 93

Section 3: Lipedema 97

What Is Lipedema? 99

Lipedema Diagnosis 101

Pathophysiology 110

The Emotional Aspects of Lipedema 112

Weight Loss, the BMI Index, and Lipedema 114

Diet and Nutrition 116

Compression Therapy 117

Other Therapies 120

The Role of Liposuction in Lipedema 121

Why Lipedema Liposuction Differs from Cosmetic Liposuction 125

Patterns of Fibrosis in Lipedema 127

Preoperative Considerations 129

The Anesthetic Approach to Lipedema 131

Various Surgical Approaches to Lipedema 133

The Tools for Lipedema Liposuction Surgery 136

CONTENTS

The Process of Liposuction for Lipedema Patients 138

Surgical Tightening 144

Lipedema, Varicose Veins, and Venous Insufficiency 147

Orthopedic Surgery and Lipedema 148

Postoperative Recovery for Lipedema Patients 149

The Long-Term Prevention of Lipedema 153

About the Author 157

Notes 161

PREFACE

Early on in my medical career, I made the decision to master the art of liposculpture. Liposuction is so much more than just sucking out fat. From the beginning, the surgery mesmerized me as being different from any other surgery. I quickly developed a profound respect and appreciation of the artistry required. As the focus of my practice, I have performed over twelve thousand liposuction surgeries over more than twenty-five years, and I have earned national and international recognition in both public and medical circles as a master of liposuction. In writing this book I hope to share my philosophies and advanced techniques to empower both my fellow surgeons and patients.

I have always been one to care a lot about the guidance of patients. My philosophy is to guide by empowering with knowledge—the more knowledge you have, the better decisions you make. When it comes to cosmetic medicine, I continue to see a trend where patients are not doing their due diligence in learning enough about their procedure of choice.

Traditional media outlets and social media have provided a powerful illusion regarding cosmetic medicine. Gone are the days of receiving a trusted referral from a friend or doctor; instead, we make decisions based on information gained from online sources. The media loves to represent the newest technologies, and we are overwhelmed by information and choices—when first and foremost the most significant decision a patient can make is the choice of the surgeon they are trusting to take them through their journey.

Furthermore, social media has developed a concerning dichotomy where a doctor can represent themselves as an expert simply by having a large number of followers. There is also an alarming amount of price-driven marketing in the realm of cosmetic medicine. In sharing my knowledge I hope I will empower you to ask the right questions, and in turn make the right choices regarding liposuction and your surgeon.

This book is divided into three sections: Cosmetic Liposuction, Revision Liposuction, and Lipedema. Regardless of your objectives and needs, I hope to demystify liposuction so you can understand the different approaches, strategies, tools, and technologies to obtain a superior result.

—David Amron, MD

INTRODUCTION

Liposuction is a contouring and sculpting procedure not that dissimilar to sculpting a beautiful piece of artwork. As with any cosmetic surgery, liposuction surgery is extremely dependent on the experience and skills of the surgeon. Liposuction is a balancing procedure, and unless comprehensive evaluation is performed by the surgeon, a patient may be thrown permanently out of proportion.

This book shares the knowledge, skills, and philosophies I have developed in a career spanning over twenty-five years focused on sculpting the human body. It provides information on cosmetic liposuction, revision liposuction, and the treatment of the disease Lipedema with liposuction. Because this book is intended not only for patients, I have also included clinical pearls for my fellow surgeons.

My advanced approach to liposculpture surgery has been honed and refined over twelve thousand surgeries. This book delves into the principles of design, engineering, artistry, and specific unique techniques I have developed in a career dedicated to one procedure: liposculpture surgery.

I strongly encourage patients to learn as much as possible and be discerning in making decisions prior to any surgery. Do not be impulsive; take the time to educate yourself. I understand that, as a patient, it can be difficult for you to sort through the aggressive, often hyped-up, and confusing marketing. But with time, patience, and good judgment you will increase your chances of finding the right surgeon to perform your surgery and make you happy with an optimal result.

SCIENCE, ARTISTRY, ENGINEERING, DESIGN

Many years ago, I was featured on a BBC special hosted by British-American documentary filmmaker Louis Theroux. While I was being filmed performing liposuction, I was asked by Mr. Theroux in the operating room, "Do you think what you do is more science or artistry?"

I pondered for several seconds and answered, "Well, liposuction is certainly based on science, but at some point, it actually becomes more about the artistry."

More recently, an astute patient of mine, who asked many questions about my process and technique, told me that they thought of me as an engineer. Well, that also does fit. Engineering is the application of science to solve problems. Good engineers make designs that work well. This is true with any successful process and applies to surgical procedures as well. They must be based on science, be engineered and designed properly, and have refined artistry. This certainly applies to achieving consistently great results for such a technically challenging and artistic procedure as liposculpture surgery.

Finally, surgery—and especially liposuction surgery—takes immense technical prowess and is physically demanding. It also requires grace and intense focus to perfect the result.

THE HISTORY OF LIPOSUCTION

The first known use of suction to remove fat from the body was performed by French surgeon Charles Dujarier in the 1920s. The development of modern liposuction is credited to Italian gynecologist Dr. Giorgio Fischer who, in 1974, invented a blunt hollow surgical instrument called a cannula that allowed for the creation of tunnels between major blood vessels of the body while sucking out fat. These early liposuction surgeries were performed almost exclusively under general anesthesia and were plagued by adverse side effects including excessive bleeding, prolonged recovery time, and skin irregularities.

In 1978, two French surgeons, Illouz and Fournier, developed a new liposuction technique with the injection of local anesthesia, saline, distilled water, epinephrine, and hyaluronidase, which helped dissolve tissue holding the fat prior to suctioning. This technique—known as the wet technique—was introduced to the United States by several American dermatologists who had been to France to observe Illouz.

Liposuction continued to increase in popularity in the early 1980s until 1985, when Dr. Jeffrey A. Klein, a California dermatologic surgeon, performed his first liposuction procedure using local anesthesia. Known as the tumescent technique, Dr. Klein infiltrated large amounts of dilute lidocaine and epinephrine into the tissue until the area was swollen (tumescent), allowing the patient to have liposuction performed totally by local anesthesia, with increased safety and less bleeding. Dr. Klein presented his new technique to the medical community at the second World Congress on Liposuction, sponsored by the American Academy of Cosmetic Surgery, in 1986. This new tumescent technique also led to the development and use of smaller cannulas for better results.

The next significant development in liposuction occurred with the introduction of energy-based devices. In 2002, VASER liposuction, using the power of ultrasonic vibration, or "vibration amplification of sound energy at resonance" (VASER), was introduced. Used in conjunction with tumescent liquid, VASER liposuction uses ultrasonic probes inserted into the fatty tissue, where ultrasound high-frequency vibrations break up the fat cells and emulsify the tumescent fluid for removal using a small cannula.

In 2006, laser was introduced for tumescent liposuction. Called SmartLipo®, it was developed by the medical device company Cynosure and used laser energy to melt or liquefy fat deposits for the gentle suction and removal by small cannulas. The heat from the laser had the possible added benefit of potential skin tightening.

Numerous other surgical tools have followed, including Cellfina®, and VASERsmooth® to target cellulite, and more recently, the radio-frequency device BodyTite®, and superheated helium gas Renuvion® for skin tightening.

Over the years, as liposuction has become more refined with experience, safety, patient selection, preoperative assessment, fluid management, proper technique, and overall patient care, its popularity has increased.

In the last decade, liposuction procedures have risen by approximately 25 percent from 198,251 in 2009 to 265,209 in 2019.[i] In 2019, The American Society of Plastic Surgeons ranked liposuction as the second most popular surgical procedure in the United States, behind breast augmentation, with over 265,209 liposuction procedures performed—up by 3 percent from 2018.[ii]

Paired with a wheelhouse of available tools, today's surgeon can combine techniques to yield superior body contouring results.

UNDERSTANDING THE ROLE OF LIPOSUCTION

The role of liposuction is often misunderstood by both the patient and surgeon. I have spent the past twenty-five years fine-tuning my approach and have a particular philosophy for what constitutes a good candidate for liposuction. Liposuction is so much more than just sucking out or melting as much fat as possible. Despite what a patient may request in their consultation or the mistaken goals of a surgeon, this approach will more often than not lead to a poor result.

When I consult with a patient, I am evaluating their case from a number of different perspectives. I don't go into my consultation and simply ask what they would like to treat or what they are here for. Instead, I evaluate the entire body from the neck down to the feet, from all angles, and I consider the following three factors: disproportion, weight, and laxity.

Disproportion: Is the Patient Carrying Fat Disproportionately throughout Their Body?

Twenty years ago, I was featured on the TODAY show with the perfect candidate for liposuction: an 18-year-old, 110-pound patient. Sounds unreasonable but bear with me. The patient's mother was also on the show, and both mother and daughter shared a genetic disproportion of a thin, bony upper body with large outer thigh "saddlebags" that were significantly disproportionate to the rest of the body. This is an example of the ideal patient: regardless of weight fluctuations, the areas of disproportion do not change. These are the areas of fat that are stubborn and do not change regardless of diet or exercise.

Weight: Is the Patient Overweight?

I have never been a fan of BMI (body mass index) measurements as they relate to liposuction. The BMI scale was developed in the early 1800s as an index to categorize patients according to their height and weight. As we will discuss later in this book, it is often erroneously used to simply place patients into an obese category, when in reality, they are primarily disproportionate. A BMI measurement can signify a patient who may be at a greater surgical risk, but it is often used in bariatric weight loss surgery as the major qualifying factor.

Unfortunately, the BMI does not differentiate a body that is disproportionate. You may have a high BMI caused by disproportion, when in fact you're not overweight. Liposuction is not a weight loss technique, and if the patient is significantly overweight but in proportion, other strategies such as diet, weight loss medications, Lap-Band® surgery, or bypass surgeries may need to be considered first.

Laxity: Is There Laxity in the Treatment Area?

Patients will often grab an area of their body they dislike and wiggle and shake it around, which always leads me to ask what they would call the tissue they are grabbing on to. The first answer is always fat. The second answer is skin. But there is actually something else at play: potential laxity of the skin and underlying muscles. As we age, muscles can loosen. A good example is diastasis recti, which occurs in women after childbirth. This is where the muscles of the abdomen have stretched and separated. A patient with this concern may think she needs liposuction but instead requires an abdominoplasty (or tummy tuck surgery) to repair the muscle laxity and excess lax skin.

Intramuscular Fat

Liposuction is not the treatment for intramuscular fat. To understand intramuscular fat, a good analogy is the marbling in an expensive steak, like Wagyu beef. The fat is intertwined between the muscle fibers and can only be addressed through weight loss, good nutrition, and exercise. Whereas the subcutaneous fat that sits below the skin and above the muscle is ideal for removal by liposuction.

So, whenever a patient grabs a full, loose area and quickly calls it fat, I immediately take the opportunity to correct them. They should call what they are grabbing flab. Flab is loose, soft tissue that contains skin, the fat under the skin (subcutaneous fat), and potentially loose muscle. Liposuction targets only subcutaneous fat.

Visceral Fat

Liposuction is also not the solution to reducing visceral fat. Visceral fat is the fat within the abdominal cavity. Liposuction surgery removes subcutaneous fat. Visceral fat must be addressed by weight loss strategies such as diet and exercise, glucagon-like peptide 1 (GLP-1) agonists such as Wegovy®, Mounjaro®, or Ozempic®, or possibly weight loss surgery. Once in a while I will see a patient that is overweight with a very protuberant belly but almost no subcutaneous fat wanting liposuction. On examination it becomes clear that the fullness of the abdomen is primarily or exclusively visceral fat. This patient needs to simply lose weight with one or more of the strategies listed above and is not a candidate for liposuction surgery.

THE "COSMETIC UNIT" AND THE CIRCUMFERENTIAL APPROACH

In my decades of performing liposuction, I have come to realize the importance of looking at the body holistically for "balance and proportion". Instead of treating a single area with liposuction (which doesn't necessarily provide the best outcome), I look at the body from the standpoint of respecting what I call the "cosmetic unit". To give you an idea of what a "cosmetic unit" is, you can think of the neck, torso, arms, thighs, and lower legs as individual "cosmetic units".

In this chapter I will delve into each of these "cosmetic units" to provide you with a better understanding of how I am able to achieve superior surgical outcomes by respecting these units.

When patients consult with me, I spend time educating them on the "cosmetic unit" that encapsulates their area of concern. It is important for a patient to listen to their surgeon's understanding of their body and how a superior result is achieved by adjusting proportions and balance in the entire cosmetic area.

Every patient comes in with at least one area of their body they dislike, but the body should be observed and treated as a whole.

Neck

Starting at the top of the body, the "cosmetic unit" of the neck begins from ear to ear at the jawline and ends at the clavicles. Traditional liposuction techniques for the submental (or, more commonly, double chin) area, focus only on treating the obvious fullness in the central neck area. This can cause the untreated areas of the lateral neck to hang. My approach for the neck is to treat the area as its own singular "cosmetic unit", so it retracts back evenly, which is paramount for an area that is often the first to show age associated laxity.

Torso

Our next "cosmetic unit" is the torso, which varies slightly for women and men. For women, the torso should be looked at in its entirety and involves everything other than the breasts. The female torso "cosmetic unit" begins underneath the breasts, encompassing the axillae (armpits), carrying all the way down to the pubic area, including the hips and flanks, and ending circumferentially at the tailbone. When performing liposuction on the torso, the entire "cosmetic unit" must be considered, or you run the risk of creating disproportion in the untreated areas of the "cosmetic unit", as well as looseness and laxity in any untreated area.

In men, the chest may be considered its own "cosmetic unit" to treat gynecomastia, which is an increase in the amount of subcutaneous fat and breast gland tissue. Alternatively, it may also be included as part of the entire torso "cosmetic unit".

Arms

The arms are a common area of frustration for women, particularly the upper arm area. This "cosmetic unit" begins at the shoulders and axillae and ends at the elbows. In Lipedema patients, the entire arm down to the wrist is considered a "cosmetic unit".

Thighs

As we continue down the body, the thighs are another "cosmetic unit". Fullness in the outer thigh area (the "saddlebags") may need to be addressed, or it could be the upper outer and inner thigh, or the entire inner thigh region down to the knee. Many patients—and especially Lipedema patients—experience fullness in their entire thigh "cosmetic unit". The ultimate goal when treating the thighs is to look at them in a three-dimensional manner and treat circumferentially to create the right balance and shape.

The "Cosmetic Units":

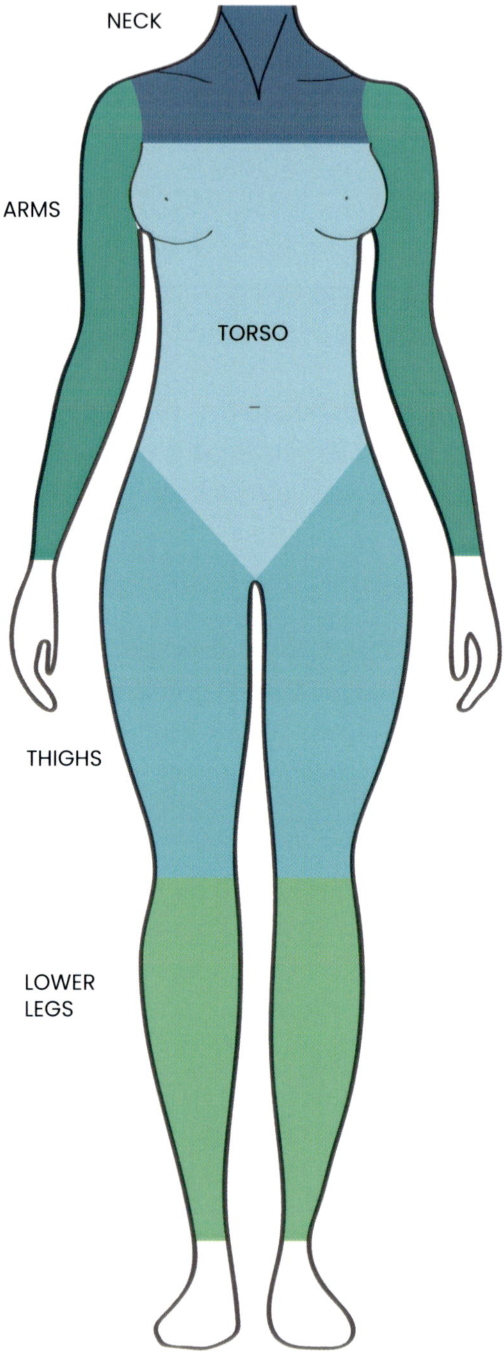

Lower Legs (Calves and Ankles)

The last "cosmetic unit" of the body is the lower legs, which includes the calves and ankles. This is an area that should never be broken up into portions and should be blended in its entirety as one circumferential "cosmetic unit".

Much of the revision work I perform as a liposuction surgeon occurs because the previous surgeon did not consider the "cosmetic unit" in its entirety. For example, when I began practicing liposuction over twenty-five years ago, I saw many patients who were unhappy with their results, especially in the tricky areas of the calves and ankles. This was because their previous surgeons had only treated bits and pieces of the calves and ankles. Their surgeons did not understand that to shape an entire area, like the lower legs, you must visualize it as a curved three-dimensional "cosmetic unit" that begins at the knee and ends at the ankle.

This piecemeal approach to liposuction also became obvious in my patients seeking torso revision work. Many would complain of the disproportionate way their body was storing fat in their mid to upper back after having liposuction done on their abdomen or flanks. These revision surgeries could have been completely avoided if the initial surgeon had respected and addressed the entire "cosmetic unit".

This leads to a common misconception, with a partial truth. Many patients think they will gain more weight in another area after receiving liposuction. Instead, this secondary response is likely caused by not treating the entire cosmetic area in the first place. Fat cells are "storage units." If you take fat cells away from an area, the body rebalances itself, leading to a disproportionate redistribution of fat. It is reasonable to prioritize and target those most disproportionate areas first, but ultimately, without synergistically treating the entire "cosmetic unit", disproportion will inevitably be created.

SECTION 1: COSMETIC LIPOSUCTION

THE THREE-DIMENSIONAL CIRCUMFERENTIAL APPROACH

Building upon the idea of the "cosmetic unit" is the circumferential approach. This is a key point in understanding the philosophy behind addressing disproportion and creating balance with liposuction. The "cosmetic unit" must be viewed as a curved three-dimensional object, and many times, must be sculpted circumferentially. Over twenty years ago, I developed a three-dimensional circumferential approach respecting these "cosmetic units" that is increasingly being appreciated as an advanced form of liposculpture surgery.

Many of the problems I see that had been created by other surgeons were the result of not blending an area in a three-dimensional manner. The body is three-dimensional with curves and roundness. When an area is treated without appropriate blending, it can create an unnatural, flat appearance.

For example, if a patient has had aggressive liposuction performed to the central abdomen, but they actually have fat and fullness around their entire waist area going all the way back to the spine, then treating only the abdomen will create disproportion in the "cosmetic unit". This leads to an unbalanced three-dimensional look from every angle of the patient's body.

The torso should often be approached in a circumferential manner, particularly in women, to provide the right type of shape and contour. Skin laxity should also be considered with the circumferential approach, to aid in the even contraction of lax skin.

Similarly, in the treatment of thighs, I unfortunately often see aggressive treatment of the outer thighs, leading to a flattened, masculine appearance that could have been simply avoided by performing the right type of three-dimensional blending throughout the "cosmetic unit".

The curves of the calves and ankles must also be approached in a three-dimensional circumferential fashion, as the rapid curvature of the lower legs can make an unblended appearance far more obvious.

Ironically, the instruments used to perform liposuction on the curves of the body are straight. This is where the importance of patient positioning comes into play during surgery. Correct positioning aids in the three-dimensional contouring of the body, leading to a superior result.

Below: Patient and surgeon positioning for anterior thigh

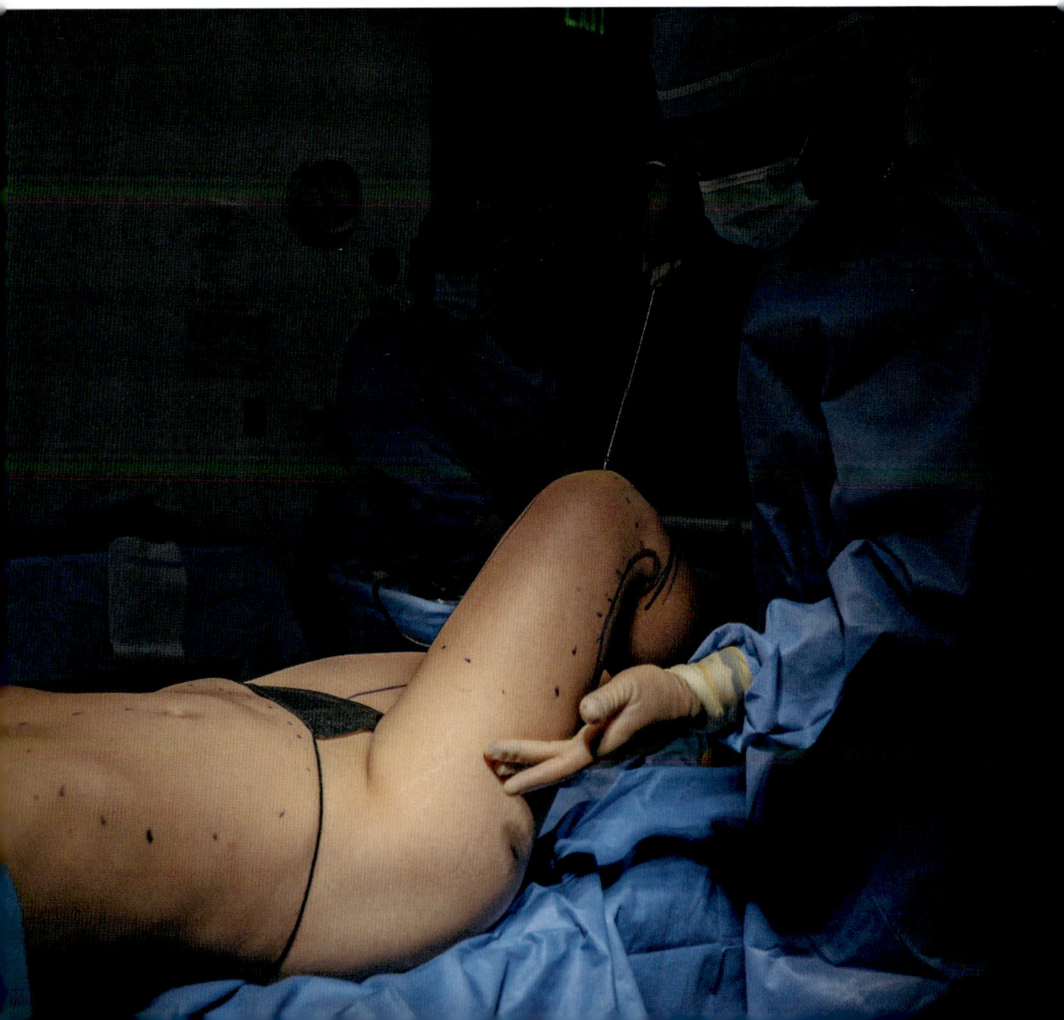

The Circumferential Approach:

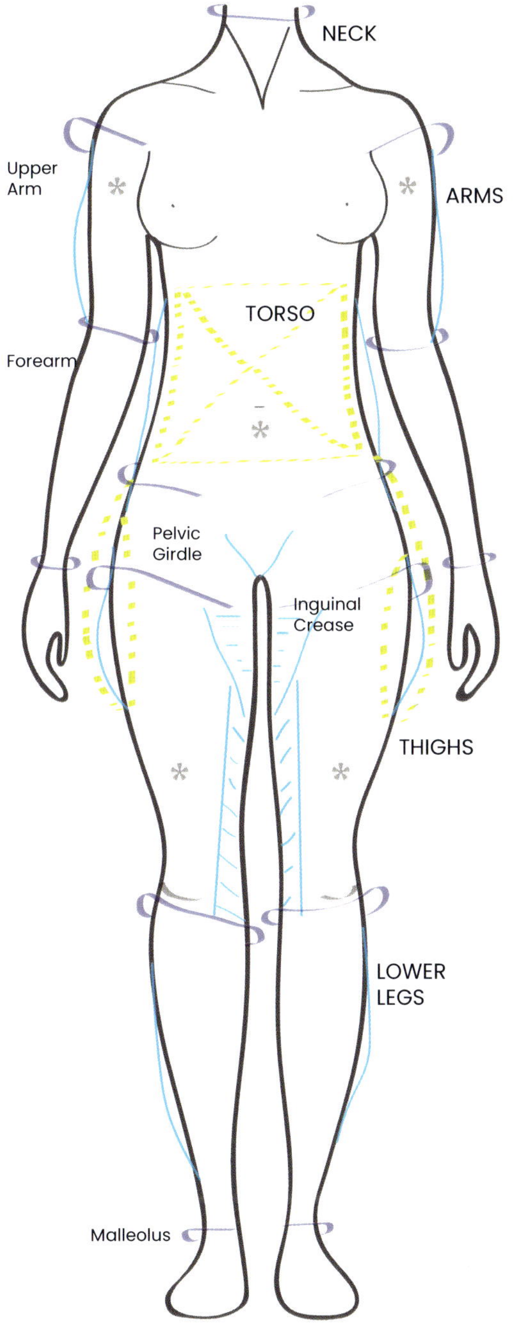

Performing liposuction three-dimensionally is a technically challenging procedure that daunts many surgeons. It takes a lot of understanding and technical know-how of the importance of body positioning and anesthetic considerations.

When the three-dimensional circumferential approach is successfully applied to each "cosmetic unit", it leads to superior, more natural-looking outcomes, without the need for subsequent revision surgeries.

NATURAL DEF LIPO

Before discussing my technique called Natural Def Lipo, I want to first educate you on High-Definition Liposuction—a commonly represented ultrasound-assisted liposuction procedure that was developed approximately twenty years ago.

High-Definition Liposuction is an extreme liposculpting technique used to expose and highlight muscle groups. With the right lighting, results can look good in a photograph but can often appear unnatural in person.

Commonly referred to as "ab sculpting," High-Definition Liposuction of the abdomen involves aggressively creating scars under the dermis so that the skin will contract unevenly to replicate the appearance of a muscle bundle. This "ab etching" can mimic the appearance of a carved, defined "six-pack" abdomen. Unfortunately, over time there is a risk of areas settling and the scar tissue tethering the skin unevenly, creating an unnatural appearance.

There are good candidates for High-Definition Liposuction, but in my experience, women are very rarely good candidates. My technique for Natural Def Lipo is a more moderate approach that thins the fat in a uniform way across the entire "cosmetic unit" to show the natural musculature underneath. This technique allows the skin to retract evenly, providing a superior, more natural-looking result.

What's the Difference?

High-Definition Liposuction	Natural Def Lipo
Fat may be removed too aggressively	Uniform and even removal of fat respecting the skin elasticity
Artificial definition by creating ab-etching scars underneath the skin	Follows the plane of muscle that already exists
Candidates include a small minority of patients	Candidates include a majority of patients with a range of body types
Commonly only addresses isolated parts of the "cosmetic unit"	Addresses the "cosmetic unit" circumferentially
Post-op nausea from general anesthesia	Avoids risks of general anesthesia

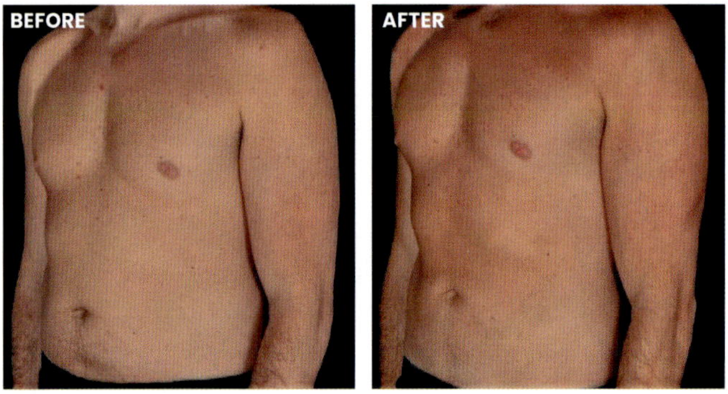

Above: Abdomen Natural Def Lipo results

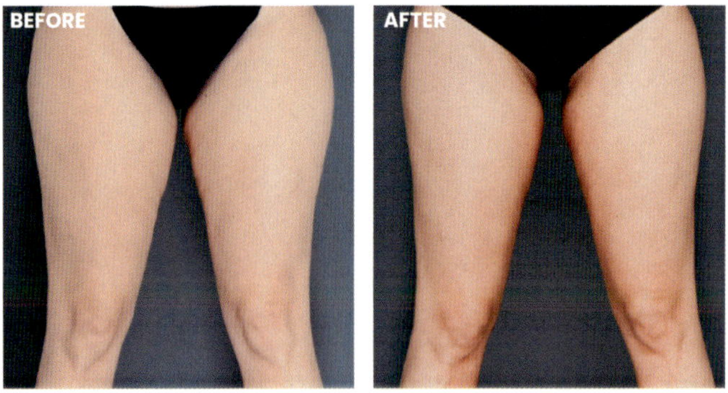

Above: Thigh Natural Def Lipo results

THE ANESTHETIC APPROACH

When first introduced, liposuction was performed under general anesthesia. Historically, general anesthesia for any procedure incurs some risk, but statistically, only one in eighty thousand patients will die from general anesthesia. This mortality rate increases significantly with general anesthesia for liposuction, which shows an approximate mortality rate of one in five thousand.[iii] What causes this mortality rate in association to liposuction? There is an increased risk of deep vein thrombosis (DVT) causing pulmonary embolism (PE), as well as the risk of perforation of an organ or other vital structure under general anesthesia.

The safety profile for liposuction changed in 1986 when Dr. Jeffrey Klein introduced the tumescent liposuction technique. Tumescent liposuction is an outpatient procedure that is performed without the use of general anesthesia. It involves infiltrating a large volume of diluted local anesthesia into the fat beneath the skin. This causes the targeted area to become swollen and firm (tumescent), minimizing surgical blood loss and replacing the need for general anesthesia.

Typically, in the United States, you will find two distinct groups of surgeons performing liposuction using different anesthetic approaches. Plastic surgeons almost always perform liposuction under general anesthesia because they are used to operating on patients that way. The second group of surgeons are dermatologic surgeons, like me. We generally perform liposuction using tumescent local anesthesia, many times paired with twilight sedation. The patient is coherent yet comfortable throughout the procedure.

There are three distinct advantages to the tumescent liposuction technique:

1. Safety

Tumescent liposuction has proven to be safer than traditional liposuction.

2. Recovery

Tumescent liposuction is associated with reduced bleeding and bruising. The surgeon avoids trauma to the muscle or deeper structures, which reduces postoperative pain.

3. Results

When a patient is intubated under general anesthetic, the body is flaccid with loose muscle tone. This can lead to technical difficulties in sculpting—and a poor result. With the tumescent liposuction technique and twilight sedation, the patient is comfortable and can adjust their positioning and tighten their muscles, providing stability of the fat layer for precise sculpting over muscles—and superior results. This also forces the surgeon to stay in what I call the *"safe plane"*.

THE PROCESS

My surgical process consists of five steps:

Step 1: Tumescent Anesthesia

My process for performing liposuction begins with proper preparation of the tissue with tumescent anesthesia. This technique involves infiltrating a dilute solution of local anesthetic combined with epinephrine and sodium bicarbonate into the tissue until it becomes firm (tumescent) and white in color.

This is an important preparatory step as the epinephrine paired with the pressure of the fluid causes the blood vessels to constrict (known as vasoconstriction). This creates a bloodless field, which allows for a safer procedure with less bleeding, as there is significant blood stored in fat. In addition, the fluids from the tumescent anesthesia hydrodissect the treatment field by breaking open the tissue with water, helping to release and break apart the subcutaneous layer, preparing it for the next step.

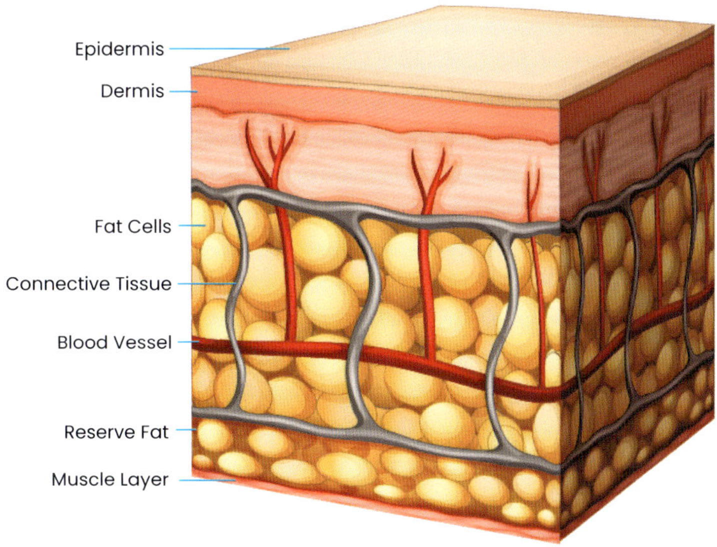

Above: A cross section diagram of skin anatomy

Pearl for the Surgeon

The safe limit of lidocaine in the subcutaneous tissues must remain below 55 milligrams per kilogram of body weight to avoid lidocaine toxicity when using tumescent anesthesia.

Step 2: Debulk and Mechanical Release

Using a vibrational device, such as power-assisted liposuction (PAL), the deeper layer of fat is precisely debulked as I release the fibrous connective tissue in the fat layer. This step is of particular importance for both revision liposuction and Lipedema patients as it helps to break up the fibrous scar tissue commonly seen in these patients.

Pearl for the Surgeon

Using a power-assisted liposuction (PAL) device with the suction setting turned off does an excellent job of pre-releasing fibrous tissue (known as vibrosuction).

Step 3: VASER

VASER liposuction uses ultrasonic vibration, or "vibration amplification of sound energy at resonance" (VASER) to further emulsify the fat layer and release the fibrous connective tissues. The emulsification of the fat creates an oily, slippery substance that protects the skin, helping it to retract in a more even fashion.

Pearl for the Surgeon

I find it better to use VASER after debulking as it more effectively targets any remaining fibrosis.

Step 4: Fine Sculpting

Fine sculpting uses smaller cannulas to perform precise sculpting of the tissue as the layer gets thinner. The cannulas are always kept parallel to the skin surface in a precise plane—I never jab into the skin from underneath. This step assists in the even contraction of the skin without causing ripples.

Pearl for the Surgeon

Preferably sculpt in the direction of skin tension lines, as this will reduce the chance of skin rippling.

Step 5: Skin Tightening

Depending on the individual, I may add the additional step of skin tightening using radio frequency BodyTite® or Renuvion®, which is ionized helium gas. This is not necessary for patients with outstanding skin elasticity and is rarely used in certain areas of the body with good skin elasticity, such as the calves and ankles.

The Five Steps of Liposculpture Surgery

1. Tumescent Anesthesia: Hydrodissect
2. Debulk: Vibrosuction
3. VASER: Emulsify
4. Fine Sculpting
5. Skin Tightening

PRECISION SCULPTING: HOW I SCULPT IN THE "SAFE PLANE"

An important aspect of my liposuction technique and philosophy is working within the "safe plane". This "safe plane" is the fat layer between the skin and the muscle. Think of it as an ocean with the sand at the bottom (the muscle) and the surface of the water (the skin) above. We want to stay parallel between those two horizontal planes when sculpting fat.

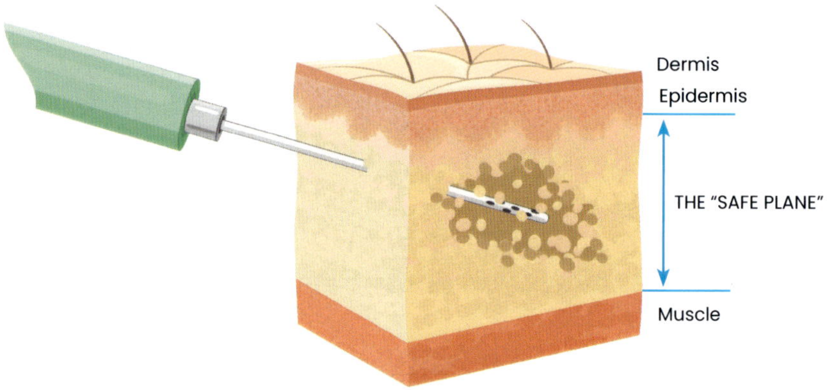

Above: A skin anatomy cross section illustrating the "safe plane" and cannula placement during liposuction surgery

Liposuction carries risks when the "safe plane" is not respected. Many years ago, I performed a revision liposuction surgery on a male patient from Texas. He told me that the orthopedic surgeon who performed his initial liposuction had perforated the aorta of a mother of three with a cannula, resulting in her death.

Many surgeons do not respect the "safe plane" and aggressively jab into wrong areas, causing unnecessary bleeding, bruising, and potential damage to organs, nerves, muscles, and tendons. This is where the benefit of local anesthesia and the tumescent technique counts. If I ever were to violate the "safe plane" during a surgery and begin to hit the muscle, my patient would very quickly jump off the tablc and lct mc know!

Liposuction is so much more than just sucking out fat. It is a detail-oriented procedure with many considerations. There should be a graceful, artistic approach to liposuction, and much of it is performed by visualizing and feeling where I am within the "safe plane". When I am sculpting with a cannula there are numerous passes I perform. I typically start deep and move from left to right in long strokes while always knowing where I am within the fat layer. This is followed by short strokes as I move up within the fat layer. I almost always crisscross in two opposite directions from above and below. In patients with Lipedema, it is especially important to release the superficial subdermal fibrosis as part of the liposculpting.

When performing liposuction in this manner you must always have respect for the skin so it will contract evenly across the treatment area. Jabbing, poking, or otherwise disrespecting the skin will increase the risk of postoperative skin irregularities. This is where a general rule regarding skin elasticity comes into play: the greater the elasticity of the skin, the more aggressive a surgeon can be with liposuction. Skin with poor elasticity will often not retract evenly, requiring a less aggressive surgical approach.

THE TOOLS

Water-Assisted Liposuction (WAL) and Tumescing

The first tool I reach for when performing surgery is a device for water-assisted liposuction, known as Body-Jet®. Water-assisted liposuction uses pressurized jets to push the tumescent fluid into the tissue. Although designed as a stand-alone system for liposuction, I utilize it in my practice as the first step to place the tumescent fluid into the tissue. Alternatively, a surgeon may use a device called the Klein pump for the same purpose, which can oftentimes be more efficient in infiltrating the tumescent fluid. Proper tumescing is an art, and it should be done gently and gracefully. Ideally, the patient should only feel mild pinching under the skin if it is performed slowly and carefully by the surgeon.

Power-Assisted Liposuction (PAL)

This tool is very popular with surgeons performing liposuction. At first, I thought of power-assisted liposuction as a tool that simply saves surgeons elbow grease to make the procedure easier for the surgeon, but it goes beyond that. Power-assisted liposuction uses vibration (similar to the vibration of a sonic toothbrush) to further release the fibrous tissue during surgery and emulsify the fat layer.

VASER Liposuction

Based on the principle of ultrasonic vibration, or "vibration amplification of sound energy at resonance," VASER liposuction uses ultrasound high-frequency vibrations to break up the fat cells and emulsify the tumescent fluid for removal. VASER is unique in its ability to target fat while leaving other important tissues intact.

SmartLipo

SmartLipo® is a laser-assisted lipolysis device that uses three laser energies: 1064, 1330, and 1440 nanometers. A thin tube containing the SmartLipo laser fiber is inserted through a small incision. The laser fiber delivers thermal energy directly to the fat cells, emulsifying the fat for easy removal with gentle suction. The heat of the laser stimulates collagen production to assist in the tightening of the skin. I treat the dense fibrous lipomas of Dercum disease with SmartLipo. Part of the SmartLipo system is called Cellulaze™, which is an energy-based device designed to release the tethering fibrous bands that cause the rippled effect of cellulite.

Renuvion

Previously known as J-Plasma®, Renuvion® is an energy-based skin-tightening device that uses ionized helium gas to contract the soft tissue below the skin with control and precision. I find Renuvion works well to uniformly contract larger treatment areas such as the circumferential torso, thighs, or upper arms.

BodyTite

BodyTite® is a skin-tightening device powered by directional radio-frequency energy that remodels and tightens tissue through fat coagulation and volumetric heating. I find BodyTite works well for specific areas, such as the "banana roll" underneath the buttocks, around the knees, and on the neck.

THE TREATMENT PLAN

When a friend or family member visits a doctor, I always ask about their doctor's diagnosis and treatment plan. Discussing a treatment plan should be an important aspect of every patient consultation. Unfortunately, in cosmetic medicine, a treatment plan is often discussed only in reference to a price quote or an estimate of fees. When I perform a consultation, I create a treatment plan based on the patient's diagnosis, evaluation, and patient value. This plan is an important strategy as it creates a path for the surgeon to follow and for the patient to understand.

When I see a patient for a consultation and evaluation, whether it's in person, or virtually with the aid of photographs, I'm developing a plan for the patient to understand and crafting my own surgical treatment plan. I am determining my exact approach for that patient, what specific areas will be treated, and whether treatment needs to consist of a single surgery or multiple surgeries. For example, when I am treating a patient with Lipedema, the treatment is almost always broken up between two, three- to four-hour surgeries. The first surgery may be done on the calves and ankles, along with the circumferential upper arms, and the second surgery may be done on the circumferential thighs. There is also a discussion of the interval of time between the surgeries, and that, of course, translates into an estimate of fees.

The consultation and evaluation allow me to educate my patient on how I will be approaching their surgery and what devices I may be using, depending on their specific concerns. I want my patient to have a very clear understanding of how the treatment will be performed. From a surgeon's perspective, there should always be a clearly laid out plan for treatment—there should never be guesswork.

When creating a treatment plan for revision work, the diagnosis is important as we may be dealing with irregularities, disproportion, and scar tissue. I discuss with the patient what devices I will use to emulsify the scar tissue and how I plan to rebalance the proportions of their body or correct abnormalities.

Pricing

Choose your surgeon first, and don't be lured by pricing strategies. I've seen many revision patients who chose their initial surgeon based on price instead of what was best for them. But price is obviously an important consideration in terms of what each patient can afford. If you are seeking multiple quotes, go with the surgeon you are confident in, even if it requires waiting until you can afford it. It's better to pay a little more to get it done right the first time instead of risking the potential expense of a more complicated revision surgery.

I see larger body contouring clinics taking almost an à la carte approach to their treatment plans by pricing treatments by areas instead of looking at the body holistically. This doesn't typically lead to a good result, as ultimately the surgeon should be making very clear recommendations instead of providing a shopping list of areas a patient may pick and choose from based on cost. This approach can often seem like a good deal, with the first treatment area being significantly discounted, but once other areas are added on, the costs can add up quickly to a bill of over thirty thousand dollars.

Pearl for the Patient

If an estimate is given for a procedure, make sure you and the surgeon are clear as to what exactly is being addressed in the surgery.

My approach to pricing is based on the complexity of treatment and the amount of time it will take for me to perform surgery. I do not price my surgeries by the area, as every patient has different needs. In my opinion, the fairest pricing follows an hourly cost and is based on how long the surgery takes. If a patient requires an additional tightening step such as Renuvion® or BodyTite®, I charge accordingly for the additional time it takes to complete that step.

There are different components the patient is paying for with liposuction surgery, including the surgeon's fee, operating room fees for the surgical center, and anesthesia. The global fee includes the surgeons professional fee, with some of that cost going toward the operating room, staff, anesthesia, and surgical supplies. I prefer to list my fees based upon the time in the operating room plus my professional fee. Anesthesia is typically a separate fee that is paid directly to the anesthesiologist. Some facilities may charge separately for laboratory tests and garments, which I don't feel is unreasonable, as this may also be rolled into the global fee. It is appropriate and fair for patients to ask what the components of their fees consist of.

As a patient, be careful of predatory pricing behaviors. Some surgeons may artificially inflate their pricing so they can go into the consultation and have the coordinator slash it down, making it appear like you're getting a deal. I've also seen surgeons and coordinators profile a patient and charge more based on the quality of their clothing, handbag, or jewelry.

I don't believe it's unreasonable for a patient to negotiate their fees. It is fair to respectfully ask if you can work with a fee. A surgeon is generally going to have to pay for the exact operating time, the anesthesia and anesthesiologist, garments, and labs, so any discounts given are typically only taken from the surgeon's professional fee.

Don't get too focused on finding a bargain. There's no bargain when things are not done well, and I'm speaking from experience with all the revision work I do. I feel badly for my revision patients as it can often take twice as much work to make things better. They had already spent a significant amount of money the first time, trusting that surgeon. Going back to that initial surgeon a second time would likely lead to a poor result. I am sensitive to my revision patients, and I try to keep the fees as low as possible, but the reality is, revision surgery is usually more complicated and time-consuming to perform.

Pearl for the Patient

Make sure the surgeon (not the consultant or patient concierge) is defining what should be done and how.

MARKINGS AND INCISION POINTS

Markings

Markings and incision points are an important aspect of liposuction, providing the surgeon with a visual understanding of how they will approach each surgery. Every surgeon has their own way of marking their patients, ranging from minimal markings to the use of complex topographic lines and different colors.

Over the years I have developed a system of marking that works for me and makes great strategic sense. Markings are an important guide because when you're on the table with a patient, they are moving around and have loose muscle tone. I mark the entire area that I am treating. For example, the upper outer thigh "saddlebag" area would have a marking at the perimeter. It may have markings within the field I'm working on, either highlighted by certain areas that show high points (like the topographical map of a mountain) or by concentric circles or x's in areas. My markings may also show an area I want to blend into with hatched lines.

When marking, I also take into consideration the perimeter of the area. For example, the "cosmetic unit" of the thighs has a huge perimeter, extending from the knee up to the groin circumferentially. I strategically divide this area into four compartments to treat: the medial compartment, the anterior compartment, the full lateral compartment, and the posterior compartment.

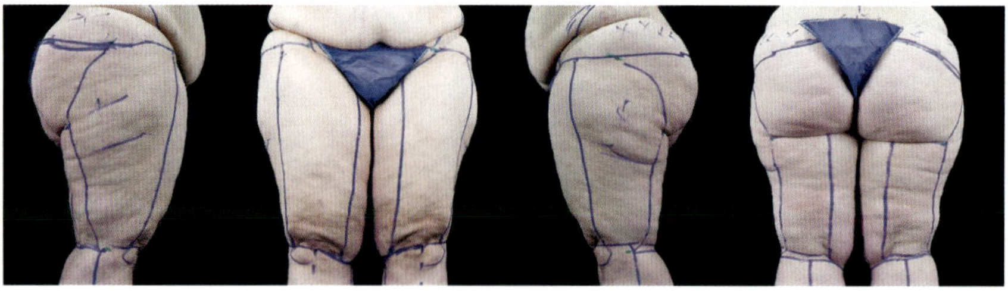

Above: Circumferential thigh markings

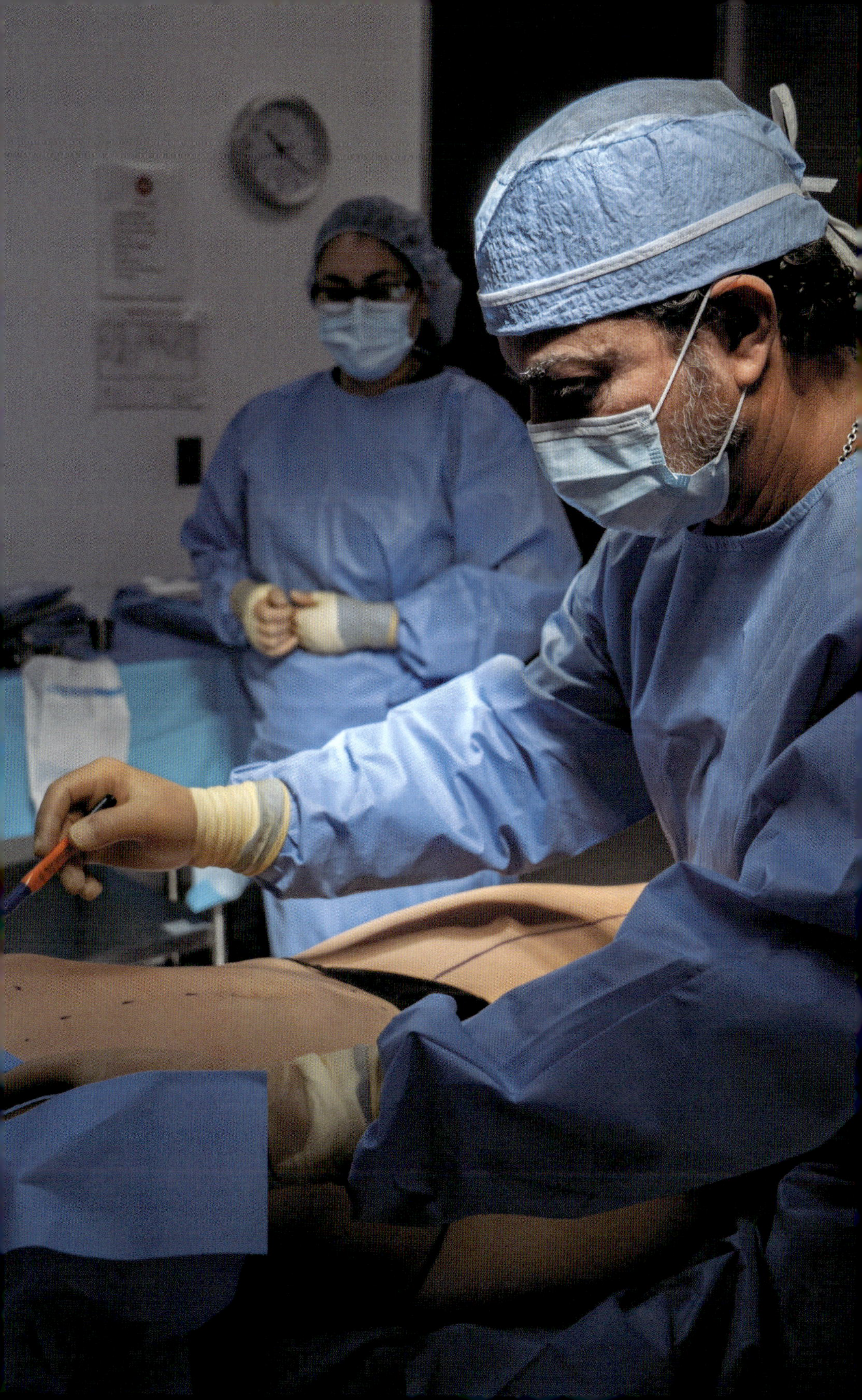

My calf and ankle markings are very different to those of most other surgeons. They are done in a triad with a lateral posterior compartment, a medial posterior compartment, and an anterior compartment. I also make a marking over the tibial area at the front of the calf so I can respect and define that area.

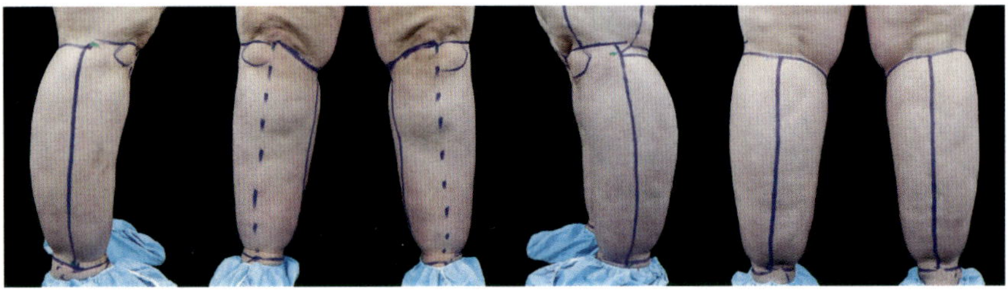

Above: Circumferential calf and ankle markings

The torso has its own exacting markings. Depending on the patient, these may include the upper and lower abdomen, along with the flank area that is being marked in a certain way, or the treatment may focus on the circumferential torso with its own set of markings. My goal with markings is to always be respectful of the entire field I am treating.

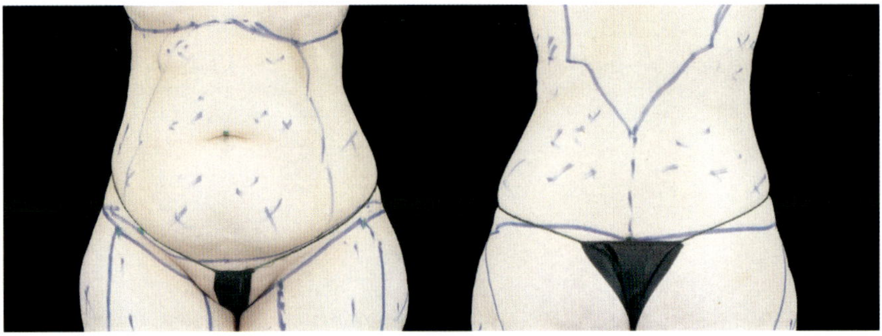

Above: Circumferential torso markings

Incision Points

During consultation, many patients express concern about the incision points and where the so-called scars are going to be. Incision points should be strategically placed and should almost never be placed within the treatment field. They should be approached from the perimeter of the field with all the work performed within it from different directions.

In my revision work I often see patients who have had their incision points placed in the middle of the field where the surgeon had been performing treatment. This doesn't make sense because you want to be able to sculpt from the outside of the field. I have also seen abdomens that have been unsuccessfully treated through a single incision at the belly button, leading to an undesired cosmetic result. This can leave a whole area around the belly button untreated because you can't physically get to it from the incision point that was placed in the belly button.

Sculpting is performed gracefully using long straight tools from strategically placed incision points. Most cannulas (including VASER cannulas) don't flex, so it is important to stay within the "safe plane" when dealing with the curvature of the body. Some surgeons may opt for curved cannulas, but in my opinion, they do not offer any advantage.

Through my years of experience I have figured out and defined exactly where every incision point should be placed to achieve the best cosmetic result for every area of the body. When I treat the circumferential torso, I place two lower incisions in the abdomen, almost in the pubic area. I will commonly make one small incision in the belly button area to be able to approach the upper abdomen from a different direction.

An important incision is placed in the axilla (underarm) area to access the entire back and waistline in a vertical direction. I discovered the benefit of this incision many years ago after seeing other surgeons treat the waistline from the middle of the back, curving around the waistline—this never works well as the rib cage gets in the way, so my approach is to have a patient lie on their side with their arms stretched above their head so that I can then reach the entire back from the axillary incision points. Another benefit to this approach is that it respects the natural tension lines in the skin. Going against natural skin tension lines can create uneven fibrous tissue formation. The more the surgeon can approach things vertically here, the better.

Below: Patient and surgeon positioning for upper back

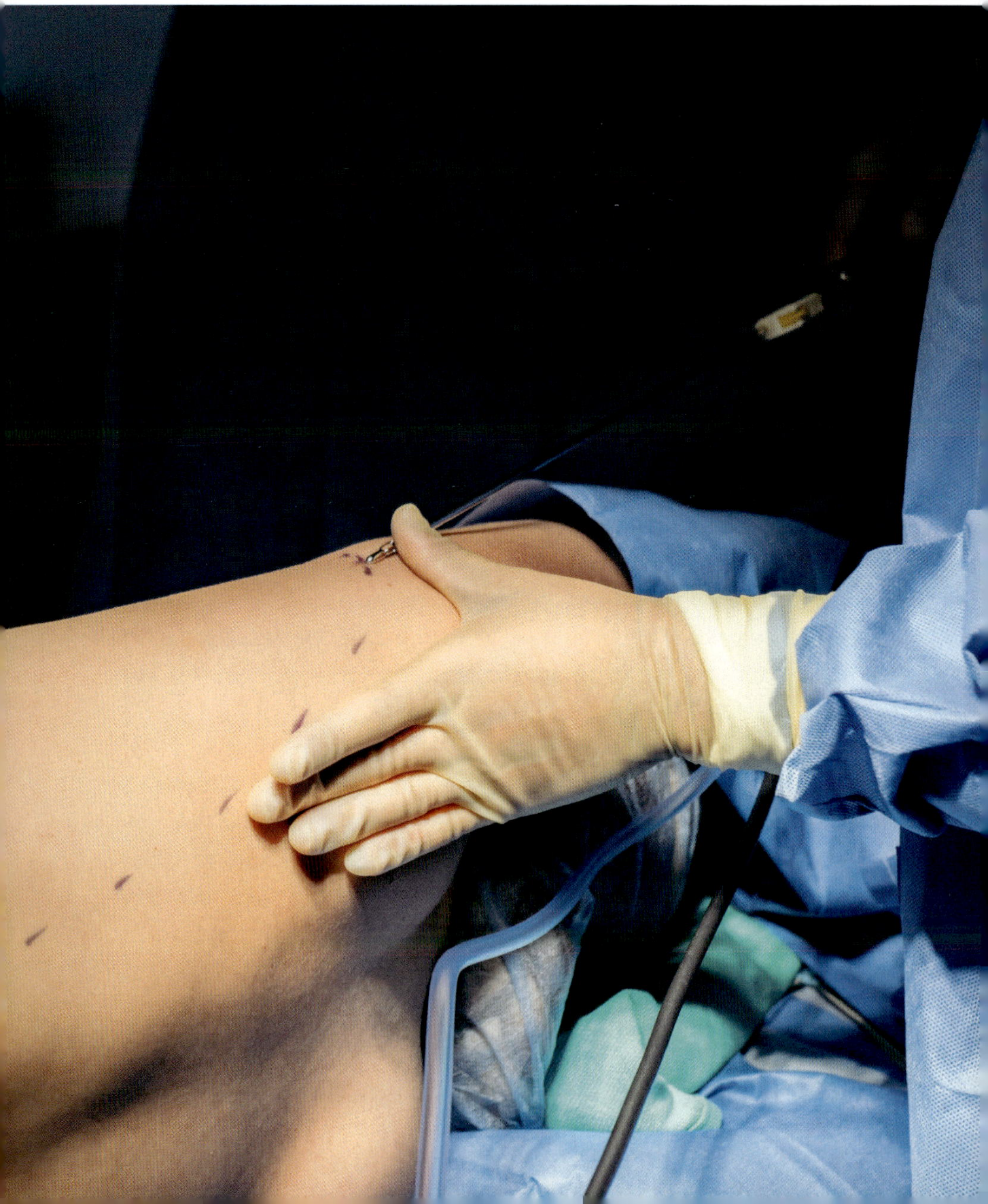

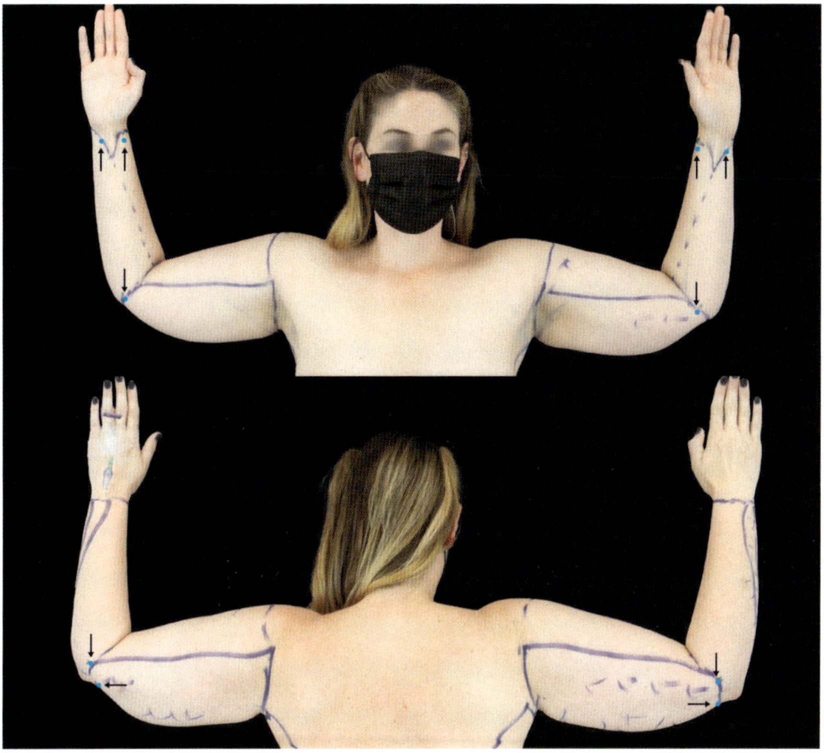

Above: Circumferential arm incision points

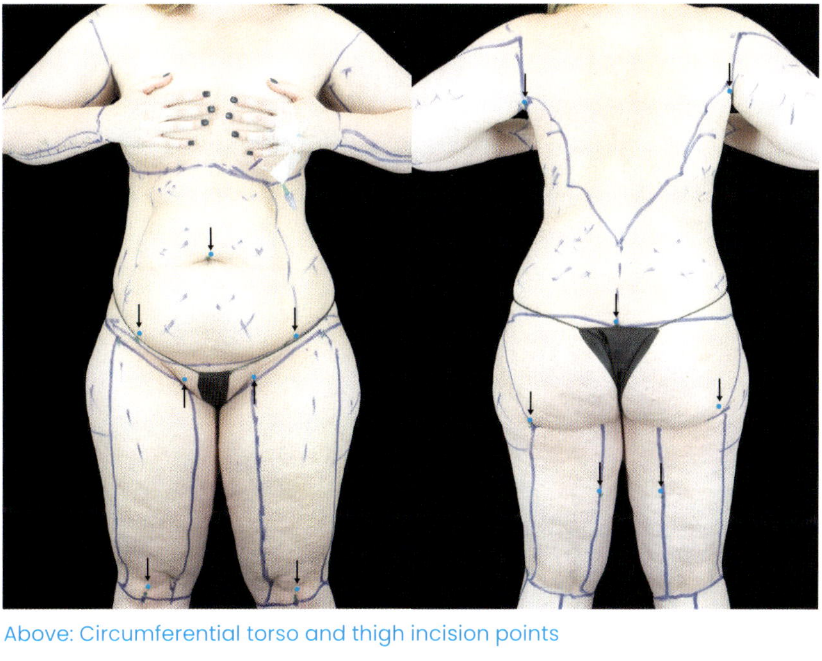

Above: Circumferential torso and thigh incision points

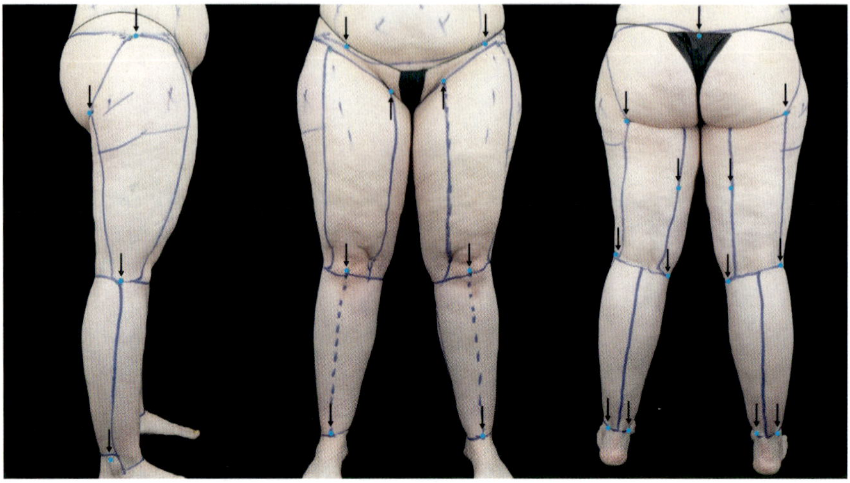

Above: Thigh, calf, and ankle incision points

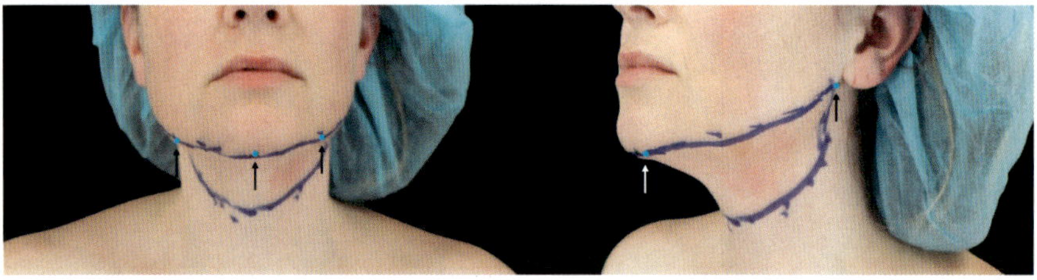

Above: Neck incision points

Correct placement of incision points for the structure of the calf and ankle is incredibly important for achieving a good result. This is an area that curves very quickly, so it can be difficult to treat these areas with long, curved instruments. The incision points for this area are always at the perimeter of the field, with two lower incision points at the lateral posterior part of the ankle and a small incision directly on top of the ankle point, which I access with the foot pointed straight down to be able to sculpt the whole tibia shinbone structure to the calf and ankle. Two upper incisions are additionally placed so I can approach from a complementary direction to shape and sculpt.

For the thighs, I make two lateral incisions to treat the entire lateral leg quadrant. I also place a small incision on top of the knee, which I then use to sculpt and shape the whole knee area and the anterior quadrant three-dimensionally. There is one incision in the upper groin area to sculpt the medial thigh quadrant, along with an inferior incision at the base of the medial knee bulge. The final incision point is in the crease underneath the buttock, to reach the posterior thigh area. With this approach the surgeon can achieve a beautiful, three-dimensionally shaped thigh area. Using fewer incision points than this will increase the chance of irregularities.

The neck area is often approached by surgeons with one central submental incision. This typically leads to an uneven retraction of the skin. For my approach, in addition to this central submental incision, I place a small incision underneath each earlobe so I can carefully approach from other directions. I find that having the patient hyperextend their neck during treatment is helpful when treating this area and respects the importance of staying in the "safe plane".

Below: Patient and surgeon positioning for lateral calf and ankle

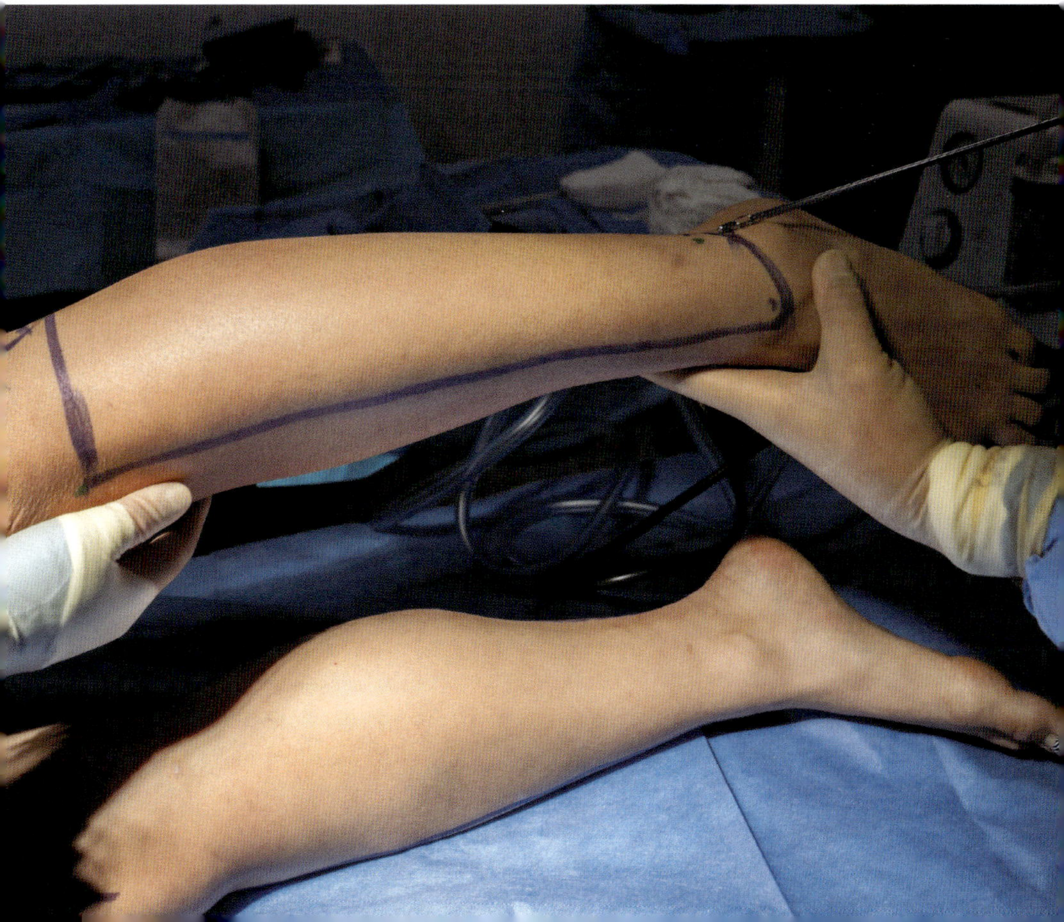

Incision Scars

Liposuction is by nature a semi-invasive procedure. Incision points need to be made to access the subcutaneous layer underneath the skin. If incision points are done well, they should be very small slits in the skin that will heal to be virtually undetectable. Some surgeons use an antiquated technique of performing a punch biopsy that removes a small ellipse of skin. I personally find this technique doesn't heal well and is unnecessary. Other surgeons create a criss-cross incision that often tends to not heal optimally.

When making my incision points, I place them in concealed areas, like the groin crease or the lower abdomen, whenever possible. Sometimes it's impossible to completely conceal an incision point, such as on the outer thigh. Incision points are placed in a horizontal or diagonal fashion depending on the area I am accessing and are always placed to respect the natural skin tension lines.

The size of an incision point ranges anywhere from two to four millimeters, with the average size being around three millimeters. Some incisions need to be enlarged for certain devices like VASER. The VASER probe uses ultrasonic energy which creates heat that can potentially burn the skin, so rubberized ports are sutured to the skin at the incision points to protect it. The surgeon should be thinking tactfully about which incision points VASER is being performed from, as it may not be necessary to access with VASER from every incision point for a good result.

Generally, most surgeons will tend to suture the incisions. Some surgeons prefer to leave the incisions open to drain. In my practice, I have found it best to lightly close the incisions without suturing them too tightly. This allows for draining, but the skin surfaces oppose so the incision heals in the best way cosmetically. I personally never use, nor ever had the need to use, drains or ports after liposuction.

There is always a potential for scarring. If the surgeon places the incision points respecting the natural skin tension lines, they should close well and heal beautifully as essentially imperceptible nicks on the skin in almost every case.

Patients who are prone to pigmentation changes to their skin may find that scars can form a bit of irritation in the area and will darken in color (known as hyperpigmentation). Lightening creams, hydroquinone, sun avoidance, and sun protection should help to lighten any changes of darkening pigmentation.

In rare cases, incisions may also become persistently red in color. This is most commonly due to irritation resulting from friction by cannulas. The irritation usually lessens over time or can be treated with a pulsed-dye vascular laser such as the VBeam® or ExcelV® to help resolve the redness.

Very rarely, an incision can form a little bump called a hypertrophic or keloid scar. Hyper means "more" and "trophic" means growth. Hypertrophic scars grow up a little bit more like a small nodule but stay within the boundary of the incision. By definition, a keloid is a scar that has grown beyond the boundary of the incision. In my experience with liposuction incision points, I have never seen an incision point form a true keloid that grows significantly beyond the incision itself. When a hypertrophic scar forms, it will generally subside with massage and/or silicone gel, or it may need to be treated with a series of dilute cortisone injections to shrink and flatten the scar nodule. This has to be performed very carefully to avoid atrophy, which is a depressed sinking of the scar.

Also in rare cases, a scar may not heal well and may form an indentation. This type of atrophic scar is usually a result of the skin retracting unevenly. If a surgeon doesn't suture an incision, it may increase the chance of an indentation forming. In my experience these indentations require surgical removal with a small elliptical excision and a few small sutures.

Overall, if liposuction is performed well and the surgeon is paying attention to how they are placing the incisions and is respecting the skin, the scars are usually imperceptible in the vast majority of patients.

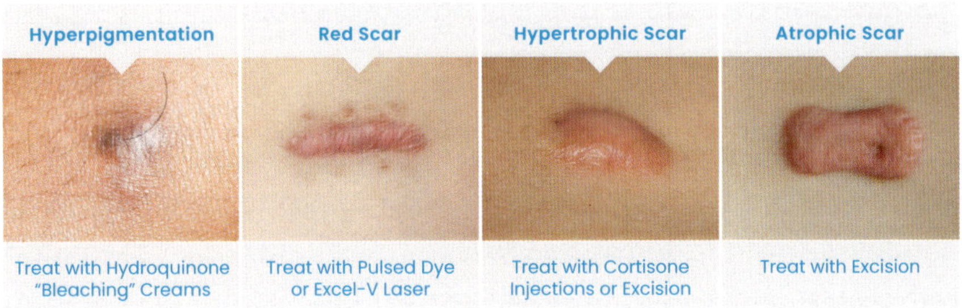

Pearl for the Surgeon

I close my incisions very lightly with one or two small 6-0 sutures—typically made of fast-absorbing gut material.

UNDERSTANDING SURFACE AREA AND SAFE LIDOCAINE LEVELS

Lidocaine is a local anesthetic drug that produces transient loss of sensory, motor, and autonomic functions when injected or applied in proximity to neural tissue.[iv] When used in tumescent fluid for liposuction, there is an important dosage calculation the surgeon must follow to ensure the patient's safety and to prevent lidocaine toxicity.

Lidocaine has a good safety margin before reaching toxic blood levels. An overdose of lidocaine, also known as lidocaine toxicity, can cause the following symptoms:

- Numbness around the mouth or of the tongue
- Metallic taste in the mouth
- Dizziness
- Tinnitus
- Blurred vision
- Restlessness, agitation, or nervousness
- Paranoia
- Muscle twitches

Large overdoses of lidocaine can result in the loss of consciousness, low blood pressure (hypotension), and slow heart rate (bradycardia).[v]

When tumescent liposuction was developed in the mid 1980s, the safe upper limit of lidocaine was 35 milligrams per kilogram of body weight. Subsequent studies and medical papers have since shown that 50 to 55 milligrams per kilogram of body weight is the safe upper limit that most surgeons should respect. In my practice, the maximum I use is 55 milligrams per kilogram of body weight.

Tumescent fluid is composed of four components: sterile saline, diluted lidocaine, epinephrine for vasoconstriction, and sodium bicarbonate to buffer the pH of the solution. Each bag of solution contains a certain amount of lidocaine and is typically mixed according to the guidelines of the Klein Solution, named for the doctor who developed tumescent liposuction. Each liter of solution contains 50 milliliters of 2 percent lidocaine (100 milligrams of lidocaine per liter), 1 milligram of epinephrine, and 10 cc of sodium bicarbonate. A full-strength bag of Klein Solution contains 1,000 milligrams of lidocaine.

To calculate how much lidocaine a patient can safely have, I will use an example of a patient who weighs 147 pounds. Their weight converts to 70 kilograms, which is multiplied by 55 milligrams of lidocaine, equaling 3,750 milligrams of lidocaine. This is their maximum safe dosage. If each liter of solution contains 1,000 milligrams of lidocaine, this patient can safely have only 3.75 liters of solution at one time during their entire procedure, otherwise they may risk lidocaine toxicity.

When undergoing liposuction under tumescent anesthesia, with or without twilight sedation, a patient may want to have their whole body treated but they can't because of the exceeding limits of lidocaine. This leads to the limiting factor of the patient's surface area. A surgeon must determine ahead of time how much surface area can be treated safely with the maximum amount of lidocaine calculated for that patient.

Depending on the treatment plan, more than one surgery may be required to remain within the safe limit of lidocaine dosage. For example, it is impossible to treat the circumferential torso and circumferential thighs together in one surgery. Instead, it may be broken up into two surgeries spaced at least forty-eight hours apart to allow the body to clear the lidocaine from its system. For Lipedema patients, I schedule surgeries one month apart to allow for adequate patient recovery time.

Liposuction performed on an intubated patient under general anesthesia is not as limiting in regard to lidocaine levels. A surgeon may do a version of a wet technique, with less fluid and less lidocaine, so there is a potential to treat larger surface areas at one time. This is not without the increased risks of more bleeding and a prolonged recovery time.

Pearl for the Surgeon

The amount of lidocaine per bag can be diluted into what I call three-quarter strength, two-thirds strength, or half strength. In my practice, I routinely use half strength, in which each liter has 500 milligrams of lidocaine, instead of 1,000 milligrams. This increases the amount of fluid I have to work with from 3.75 liters up to 7.5 liters, allowing me to stay within the safe dosage of 55 milligrams per kilogram of body weight. This gives me the ability to treat a larger surface area, such as the circumferential thighs or circumferential torso. In my experience, going below half strength may not sufficiently tumescently numb an area, causing the patient sensation and discomfort.

AMOUNT OF FAT REMOVED

Patients always want the maximum amount of fat removed, and it's commonly thought that the more fat that's removed, the better. However, this is not the case, and one of the biggest mistakes a surgeon can make is to approach liposuction from the standpoint of determining how much fat can be removed. Being overly aggressive with the removal of fat can lead to an unnatural look and can create irregularities of the skin.

I encourage patients to not be lured into thinking that more is better. Liposuction is a balancing procedure where weight, laxity, and disproportion must be considered by the surgeon. In the United States, the safe upper limit of fat removal for liposuction as an outpatient procedure is 5 liters of fat per surgery, as set by the American Society of Plastic Surgeons and the American Society for Dermatologic Surgery.

However, these are guidelines, and the surgeon should use their judgment and experience to determine what is best for each patient. For a thin patient weighing 100 pounds, a much lower guideline of 3 liters may be safer, whereas a 400-pound patient may be able to tolerate much more than 5 liters per surgery.

Another factor that can influence the amount of fat to be removed is the technique the surgeon will be using. With good vasoconstriction under the tumescent technique, more pure fat can be removed with less bleeding. On the other hand, liposuction performed under general anesthesia may need to stay within the lower limits of how much fat is removed if there is significant bleeding.

In my practice, I remove anywhere from 200 cc of fat for a small area to over 12 liters for larger areas. I will commonly exceed the 5-liter limit because I have determined that it is safe for that particular patient. In general, it's better to be more conservative than to be too aggressive, as this can create issues that may be unfixable later on.

GRAVITATIONALLY PRONE AREAS: LIPOPREVENTION

Lipoprevention is a term I have coined to help patients appreciate that liposuction has a preventative component. Besides creating "balance and proportion" in a patient's body, liposuction has a great ability to prevent laxity in certain areas of the body as a patient ages. There are certain areas of the body, in both men and women, that I consider "gravitationally prone," and these are where lipoprevention becomes an important factor.

As we age, our skin loses elasticity, causing it to droop and settle. The neck is one area that typically wants to move south and drop. The upper arms are also an area in women that commonly becomes loose. If a patient is gravitationally prone in the arm area, it is important to take care of it early while the skin elasticity is still good, because as time goes on, the skin may drop and develop into so-called bat wings. The mid to upper back area, central abdomen, and upper inner thigh are also gravitationally prone areas.

If liposuction is performed earlier (as opposed to later in life when the skin has lost too much elasticity), it can help to prevent further laxity by removing the weight on the skin that is causing it to become loose and heavy, similar to removing the weight from a sack. Having a good level of skin elasticity will help the skin to recoil after the weight has been removed.

When performing neck liposuction there is typically a good amount of skin retraction, even though the amount of fat removed may be as small as two tablespoons. Using a spatula cannula to suction the skin from underneath causes a dermal injury (or irritation that stimulates new collagen production), and in turn, skin tightening. Patients experiencing sagging of the skin on their neck, especially men, may benefit from liposuction early on to prevent needing a face- or neck-lift as they age. The addition of thermal contraction such as radio-frequency Neck-Tite™ or Renuvion® can add to the tightening.

Liposuction can create significant tightening in the abdomen area, particularly in patients with stretched skin after pregnancy, reducing the potential need for a tummy tuck. Similarly, liposuction to the arms or inner thigh areas may prevent the need for brachioplasty (arm-lift) or thighplasty (thigh-lift) surgeries.

The new collagen produced from liposuction surgery forms a sling of connective tissue, similar in composition to scar tissue. The term scar has a negative connotation, but fibrous or connective tissue is the same material as scar tissue. This connective tissue forms an even sheet that lifts and tightens, almost like a supportive "shrink-wrap" that keeps the area firm and prevents age-associated laxity post surgery.

Main Areas of Lipoprevention

- Neck
- Upper arms
- Chest (in males)
- Central abdomen
- Upper back
- Inner thighs
- Knees

SKIN ELASTICITY AND SKIN TIGHTENING

When determining a good candidate for liposuction with regard to skin laxity, I view it almost like riding a seesaw. On one side of the seesaw there is excellent skin elasticity, and on the other, poor skin elasticity. There is a point where there is too much loss of elasticity and not enough fullness, which swings that seesaw to the patient being a poor candidate for liposuction without skin excision. A patient with good fullness and skin elasticity is typically an excellent candidate.

In addition, liposuction can potentially cause more loose skin if the surgeon has poor technique. If there is too much looseness, a loss of elasticity, and not enough of a fat layer, a surgeon should reconsider performing liposuction in that area, as it may lead to irregularities and more loose, wrinkled skin.

The neck and arms are great examples to demonstrate the importance of skin elasticity in relation to achieving a good result with liposuction. Loose, thin, hanging skin may not respond well to liposuction, even with the additional use of tightening devices, such as Renuvion® or BodyTite®. This loose skin may ultimately require surgical removal.

Grading of Skin Elasticity

Good to Excellent ·······➤ Typically good skin retraction without additional tightening step

Moderate ·············➤ Typically benefit from additional tightening

Poor ··················➤ Typically better to consider surgical tightening

A brachioplasty (arm lift) can leave significant scars on the arms and should be considered only as a last option. In my practice, I believe patients should try to avoid brachioplasty, particularly if they have good or moderate elasticity. Liposuction paired with an additional skin-tightening step may yield a better result for the patient without the scarring and risks associated with a surgical lifting procedure.

Many of the patients I see in their forties or fifties may have already lost too much elasticity to make them good candidates for liposuction. But ultimately, regardless of age, if a patient has a good level of elasticity, liposuction with non-excisional skin tightening may be the better option.

Even in patients with good elasticity, if the surgeon doesn't approach the skin the correct way, it may cause more looseness and uneven skin retraction. The deeper fat layer should be debulked first using a round cannula from the bottom up. I then mechanically rasp under the surface of the skin with a flat-tipped spatula cannula to encourage even skin retraction. I avoid using round cannulas too close to the surface of the skin, as they can cause grooves and irregularities.

Ultimately, the surgeon's technique is the most important factor in achieving even skin retraction. If the surgeon is not focusing on developing that uniform fibrous connective tissue sheet to tighten, there is the potential to cause more loose skin.

Another potential risk is dropping an area by severing the fibrous tissue and support structures. The buttocks area can be prone to this concern, known as ptosis. When treating the gluteal crease ("banana roll") area, the surgeon needs to be respectful of the deeper fibrous attachments by staying perfectly in that subcutaneous layer. Going in too deeply can affect the fibrous support of the buttock, causing it to drop, which is a challenging—if not impossible—error to fix.

Pearl for the Surgeon

When liposuctioning around the gluteal crease, stay superficial to prevent dropping of the buttock (ptosis).

When thinking about skin retraction in liposuction or a surgical tightening of the abdomen, there are several factors to consider. If there is too much loss of elasticity to the skin and underlying muscle structures (which is a common concern for many women after pregnancy), liposuction may be needed first to reduce the bulk of fat, followed by a tummy tuck (abdominoplasty) to remove the excess lax skin. In the medical community there has been concern regarding increased complications when a tummy tuck is combined with liposuction in the same surgery. I recommend patients listen to the advice and guidance of their surgeons about whether they are comfortable performing both procedures at the same time or as two separate staged procedures.

There are several factors to consider with liposuction to the abdomen after pregnancy. If a person has disproportion in their abdomen, my recommendation is to treat with liposuction prior to pregnancy (while the skin is more elastic) for better retraction. In my experience, it can be preventative, eliminating the need for a tummy tuck after pregnancy, because the connective tissue formed from liposuction provides support and tends to retract more effectively after pregnancy. But if there is too much looseness of the skin, an abdominoplasty may still be required.

I have treated many patients who have had several children—including my wife, Jessica. After having our fourth child, she consulted with a plastic surgeon who recommended a tummy tuck. Even after multiple pregnancies, if there is still reasonable skin elasticity and the underlying muscle structures do not require surgical repair, liposuction with additional skin tightening may be the better, less invasive treatment option. I believe a tummy tuck should always be an absolute last resort, and for Jessica I performed liposuction with Renuvion for additional skin tightening. She had excellent improvement and avoided the scarring and repositioning of the belly button associated with a tummy tuck.

If a patient truly needs a surgical tightening procedure, I recommend they consider their options and not only consider liposuction. A surgical tightening procedure may give a better cosmetic result, but it also leaves the patient with potential unsightly scars. If a patient wants to avoid surgery and scarring, we may first attempt liposuction with a tightening step, followed by a surgical tightening procedure as a final resort.

CELLULITE

Cellulite is a phenomenon that primarily occurs in women. There are genetic and hormonal components to cellulite, and it tends to worsen as women age. Cellulite is the uneven storage of fluid in the superficial layer of fat. Fibrous septae run between the muscle and the skin in a vertical orientation, predisposing that area to store more fluid between the septae and the fat tissue. This contributes to the look of unevenness at the surface of the skin.

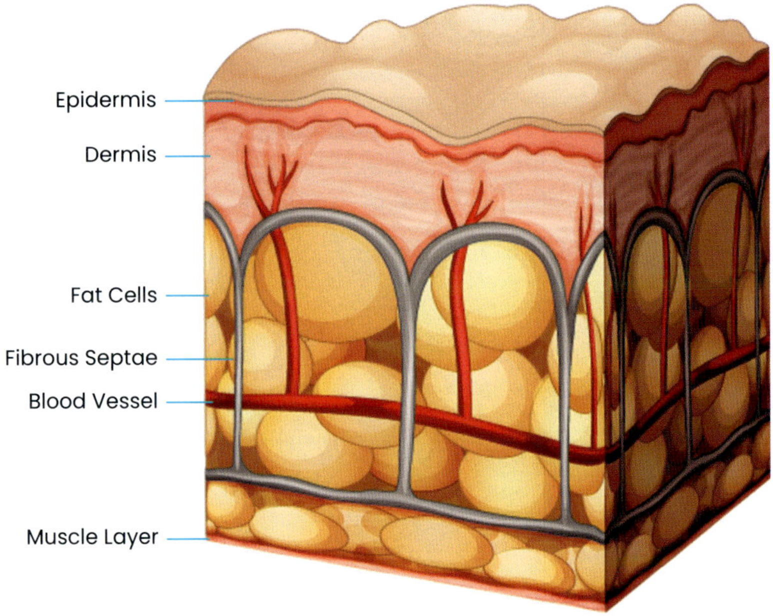

Above: A skin anatomy cross section illustrating cellulite

Cellulite can be challenging to treat. There may be improvements a woman can make to cellulite from a nutritional or hormonal standpoint, but with regard to treatments, they fall into two categories. The first is external treatment using noninvasive devices, and the second is internal treatment to improve cellulite. Liposuction itself has had a reputation for possibly making cellulite worse, and it potentially could if it is not performed with the right technique by a surgeon who is skilled in dealing with cellulite.

With regard to noninvasive treatments, there are many types of devices that can be used, and most are energy-based or energy-based suction-type devices. One of the first devices made available for the treatment of cellulite is called Endermologie®, which uses a suction-based device with energy. It can make improvements in cellulite, but most of those improvements are typically temporary. VelaShape® III is another noninvasive device that uses radio-frequency energy to externally heat the tissue to create tightening and hopefully reduce swelling. VelaShape III is FDA-cleared for the temporary reduction of the appearance of cellulite and the temporary reduction in thigh circumference. To date, there has not been a noninvasive treatment that has succeeded in making long-term changes to cellulite.

Internally, liposuction can significantly improve cellulite, when performed by a surgeon who understands cellulite and how to technically improve it. One of the techniques I have historically performed is to finish by using a flat spatula cannula under the surface of the skin to transect the fibrous bands. In my experience, this alone provides good improvement to cellulite.

The first internal energy-based liposuction device for cellulite was Cellulaze™, as part of the SmartLipo® system. Cellulaze uses laser energy to transect those fibrous bands. The ultrasonic energy of VASER, known as VASERsmooth® can also break up the fibrous bands, and in my experience is superior.

Cellfina® is a modality that uses a mechanical device to cut and release those fibrous bands, which ironically is very similar to the way I used to treat cellulite using a spatula-tipped cannula. Cellfina works well in certain areas, such as on buttock indentations, but offers no improvement to the contour of an area.

In my practice, my current treatment protocol for cellulite is to mechanically release the fibrous bands with superficial liposuction followed by VASER, which further releases the fibrous bands and emulsifies that layer of fat into an oily substance under the skin, so as the skin retracts, it does so in a smoother fashion.

Examples of Technologies to Treat Cellulite

Non-Surgical
- Endermologie
- Velashape

Surgical
- Cellulaze
- Vasersmooth
- Cellfina

COMBINING LIPOSUCTION WITH OTHER PROCEDURES

Liposuction is commonly combined with other procedures worldwide. If performed with much consideration for patient safety, it is reasonable. However, numerous studies conducted over the years have indicated that when liposuction is combined with too many other procedures, along with the operating room time becoming excessive (especially if performed under general anesthesia), the risks of morbidity and mortality significantly increase.

One must be careful when combining liposuction with other procedures. Elderly patients or patients with multiple medical problems are at higher risk for complications. Some surgeons will combine procedures such as face-lifts, rhinoplasty, breast implants, liposuction, and even tummy tucks in marathon twelve-hour surgeries. Those extensive procedures, together with general anesthesia, increase the risks for the patient.

There has been concern in the medical community over the years regarding the safety of combining extensive liposuction with abdominoplasty. When performed conservatively, it can be done safely, and it is ultimately up to the determination of the surgeon. This also matters on a patient-by-patient basis. If the liposuction is performed aggressively or circumferentially, particularly in the upper abdominal area concomitantly with abdominoplasty, this may present an increased risk.

In my practice as a liposuction specialist, I try to avoid doing extensive liposuction surgery along with many other procedures at the same time. For example, if I'm working with another surgeon, I may perform liposuction under local or tumescent anesthesia in smaller, more specific areas on a patient who is going to undergo a face-lift or rhinoplasty. Similarly, I may perform liposuction in smaller areas on a patient who is undergoing breast revision surgery. Each patient is evaluated individually based on their risk profile and the procedures being performed. A decision is then made between me and the other surgeon for how to best approach the combining of procedures in terms of patient safety and recovery. We may decide it is in the best interest of the patient to separate the procedures by days, weeks, or even months.

THE PREOPERATIVE VISIT

Ideally, every patient undergoing liposuction surgery should have medical clearance. It is up to each individual surgeon to make a determination about medical clearance and what specific laboratory tests to perform. Some surgeons don't require medical clearance on any patient, while others may require clearance on patients over a certain age, such as fifty-five. Ultimately, this should be addressed on a patient-by-patient basis. In some cases, there may be a younger patient with a complicated medical history who should have a medical clearance.

For patient safety, it is best practice to routinely get medical clearance on almost every patient undergoing liposuction surgery. Then again, if a very small area is being treated under local anesthesia, a medical clearance may not be necessary, particularly if the patient is young and without a complicated medical history. For patients who are undergoing numerous procedures at the same time, it is prudent to get medical clearance.

The medical clearance is typically performed by an internal medicine doctor, who ideally has familiarity with the patient. It's up to that doctor to determine if an EKG should be performed.

For laboratory tests, you'll find a variety of blood tests may be required. Some surgeons may require no blood tests from a patient undergoing liposuction, while others may require a large battery of blood tests, including complete chemistry panels, hematology panels, bleeding profiles, and hepatitis and HIV tests. Presently, with the COVID-19 pandemic, a COVID test should be performed on every patient.

In my individual practice, I require a complete blood count, as well as a bleeding profile called a PT and PTT. For COVID testing, every patient is tested prior to surgery, and I also require medical clearance for every patient over the age of fifty and younger patients with complicated medical conditions.

The preoperative visit gives the patient an opportunity to have any last-minute questions addressed and to review the surgical plan once again. I typically perform my preoperative visit one to two weeks before surgery on local patients. For patients who fly in from out of state, we will typically not meet for the preoperative visit until the day before surgery. Those patients will have already had their medical clearance and laboratory tests performed in their hometown, with the results sent to me. I strongly prefer to have the preoperative visit completed the day before surgery, rather than on the day of surgery.

POSTOPERATIVE CARE

Once again, each individual surgeon has their own specific patient instructions regarding recovery and healing. With liposuction surgery, patients should understand that final results will take anywhere from six and sometimes as long eighteen months, especially if we are dealing with a condition such as Lipedema.

In my practice, after surgery is completed and while the patient is still on the operating table, they are milked to assist in the drainage of the tumescent fluid and the incisions are lightly sutured with one or two small dissolving stitches. Patients are placed in compression garments and transferred to the recovery room for an hour and are given intravenous fluids to help them rehydrate.

Patients are then escorted out with their postoperative instructions in the care of a responsible friend or family member who will bring them home or to wherever they are staying. Older patients, and those with complicated medical histories, may be left in the care of a hired nurse or will stay in an aftercare facility.

Patients will typically drain from their incisions for twelve to thirty-six hours after surgery. Pads are placed over the garments at the incision sites to absorb the draining tumescent fluid, which may be blood-tinged or pinkish in color. In my patients, I have never had the need to place surgical drains.

Patients are prescribed a perioperative antibiotic that they start on the day before surgery and continue to take twice a day for seven days. Postoperative pain medications should only be taken if necessary, as they may contribute to nausea.

On the evening after the surgery, most patients are not in significant discomfort. In my practice, about 25 percent of patients take pain medication in the days following surgery.

Patients begin walking immediately after surgery but should remain in the care of a companion, especially during the first twenty-four hours. They should not be left alone during the first twenty-four hours after surgery as they may feel lightheaded and may be at risk of falling and injuring themselves. Patients are instructed to hydrate with plenty of fluids (a glass of water every hour) and to resume a normal diet.

The day after surgery, patients return to the clinic for a postoperative check. They are instructed not to shower until they have been seen through the post procedure check.

Cosmetic patients will continue to wear the surgical compression garment for two to four weeks for twenty-four hours a day, and then for another two to four weeks for twelve hours a day. Most routine daily activities, including working and continuing household responsibilities, can be resumed two to four days after surgery. Lighter exercise, such as walking, is encouraged for the first four weeks, with most patients being able to resume a normal exercise routine after that.

Approximately 25 percent of my cosmetic patients may have bruising to any significant degree. This resolves within two to three weeks. The majority of Lipedema patients will experience bruising due to their increased tendency to bruise as part of their condition.

RESULTS

The final results of liposuction may take up to a year to develop, although this could range anywhere from six months to as long as eighteen months, especially in Lipedema patients and when done in certain areas such as the calves and ankles. Patients will often return for their follow-up visit within twenty-four hours post surgery expecting to see their full result, without appreciating that there is still significant swelling.

Most patients will begin to see a very good improvement within the first month. Larger patients with a thicker fat layer of two to three inches may see a significant improvement as early as a few days post surgery. Thinner patients with a thinner layer of fat will generally take longer to see their significant improvements as there is a smaller layer of fat that has been brought down. Many times, in the recovery process, with the swelling and healing of the tissue, there is inflammation and edema that can create initial short-term swelling. Some thinner patients may actually become slightly bigger in the first month after surgery, followed by a diminution in size.

Results are important to understand. The surgeon should be providing the patients with a clear idea of their potential results as much as possible in the consultation to prepare the patient to have proper expectations.

When I discuss results with a patient, I am very careful with the words I use. When a patient uses words such as "gone" or "completely," I will alter the phrasing and talk about significant improvements in areas. Patients should always appreciate this with any cosmetic surgery. With liposuction surgery, we are often dealing with other factors, such a looseness in areas or limitation to the degree of improvement that can be made, so results should always be thought of in terms of significant improvements.

Patients should try to align themselves with the surgeon who has the greatest chance of giving them the best results and the lowest chance of creating a problem or complication. This is dependent on the individual patient and on the judgment and technical abilities of the surgeon.

Before and after photographs can be shared as a rough guide for results and for choosing the right surgeon, but I do not recommend completely trusting before and after photographs. Surgeons are going to show their best results, not their complications or poor results. Some surgeons will misleadingly alter and edit their photographs to make a result look better, so I advise patients to be very careful and skeptical when looking at before and after photographs as their only guide for choosing their surgeon.

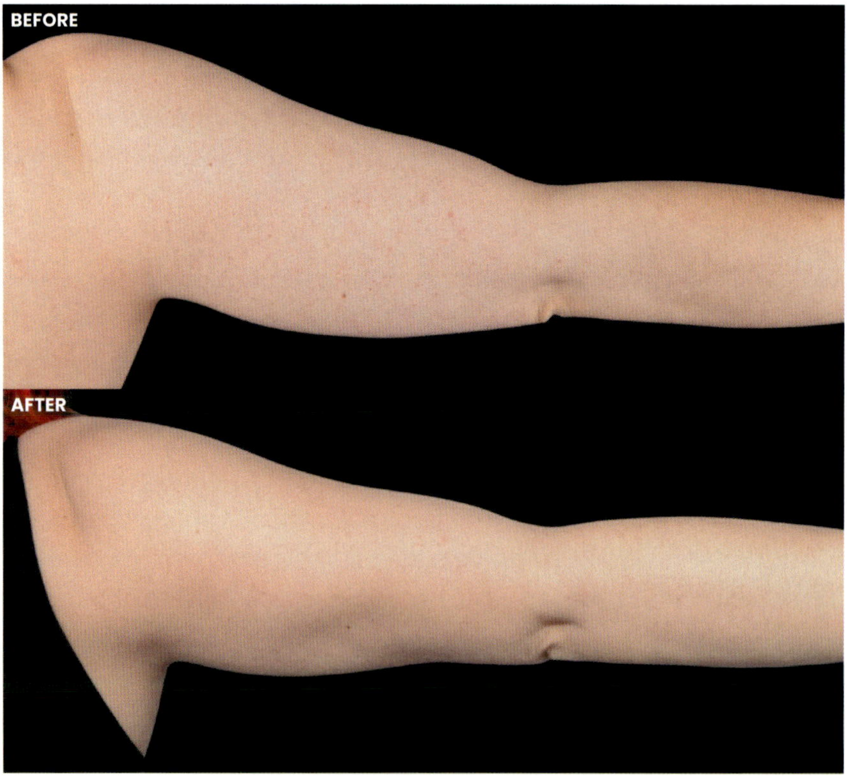

Above: Liposuction to upper arms

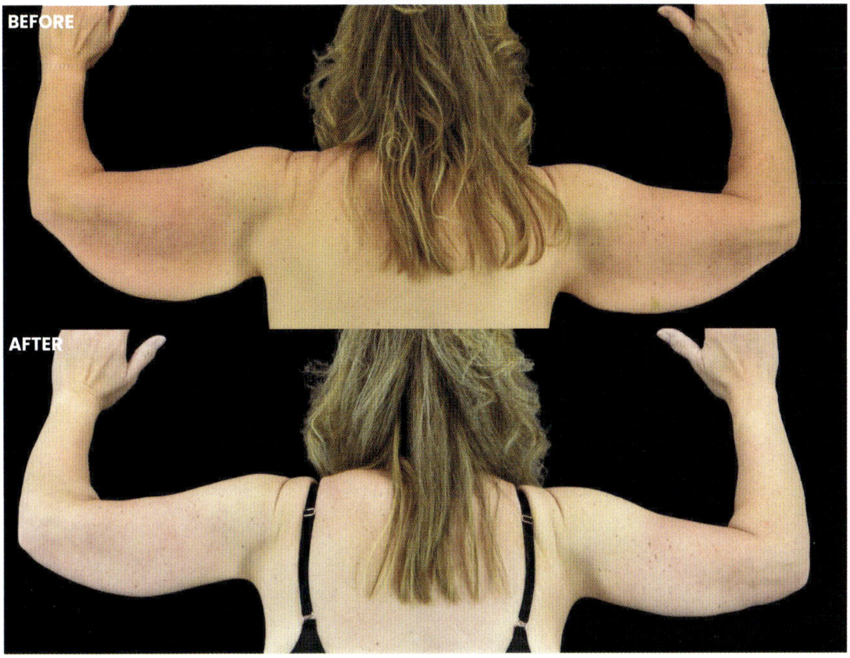

Above: Liposuction to upper arms

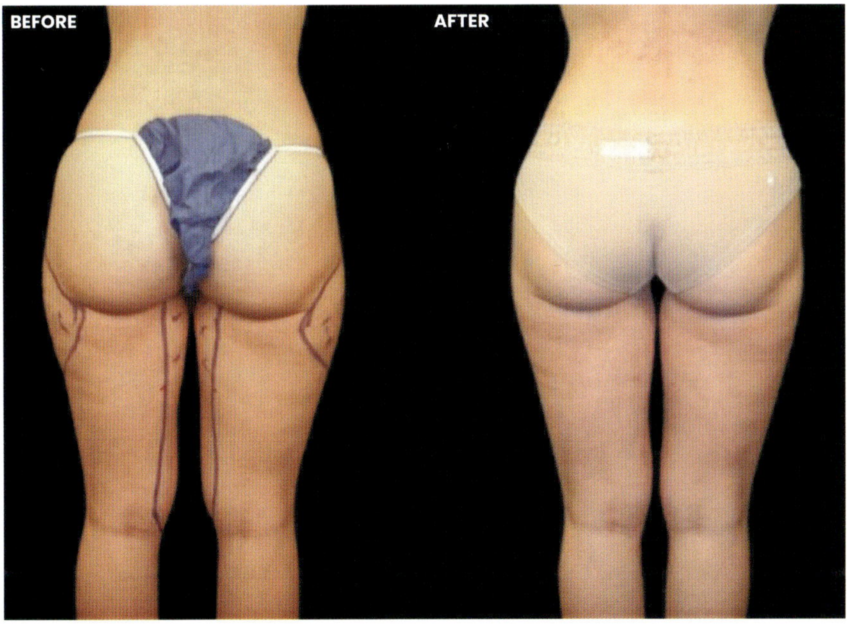

Above: Mini-liposuction to outer thighs, full inner thighs, and knees

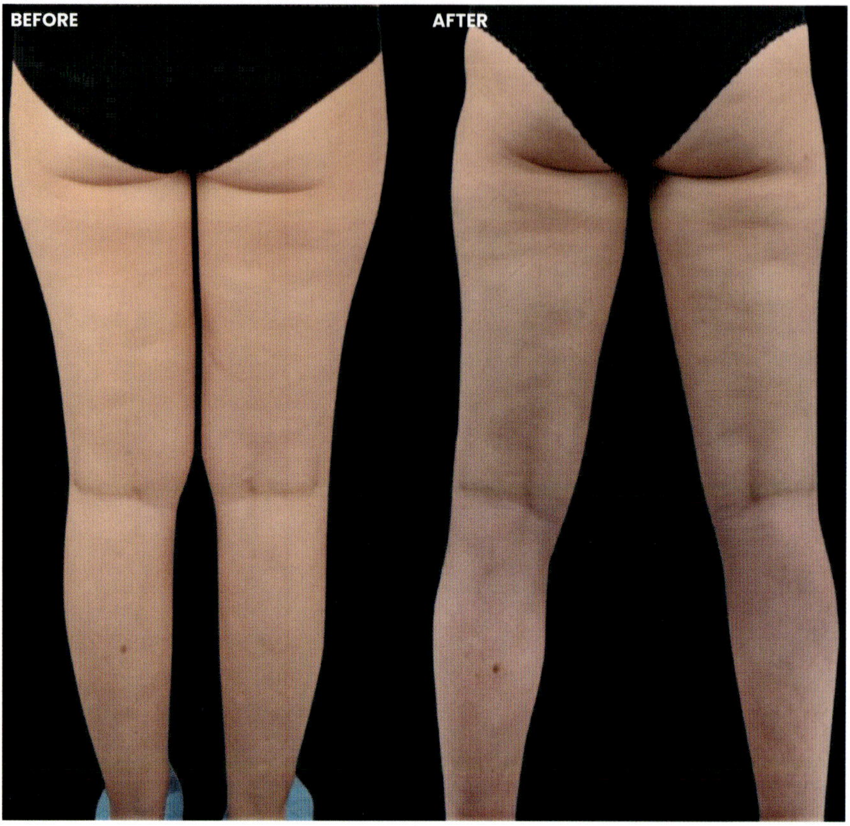

Above: Liposuction to circumferential thighs, calves, and ankles

NONINVASIVE FAT LOSS TECHNIQUES: ARE THEY WORTH IT?

The development of new noninvasive fat loss techniques has expanded rapidly over the last fifteen years. There are a lot of new technologies entering the marketplace to noninvasively contour the body. I feel that many of these technologies have been overly represented and aggressively marketed. Many of these procedures are performed by facilities or people that do not focus on or specialize in liposuction body contouring and are looking to sell packages of these procedures to anybody and everybody without truly qualifying if a noninvasive procedure is the best treatment option for the patient.

Of course, every patient wants to approach their treatment non surgically. They prefer not to do surgery and are scared about liposuction and its potential risks and complications. But I have come across an increasing number of patients who have had noninvasive body contouring techniques that did not yield a result.

Noninvasive technologies for body contouring fall into several categories. Each type of technology works slightly differently, by either heating or freezing fat cells to eliminate them from the body. One of the first that was approved by the FDA in the United States was CoolSculpting®.

CoolSculpting

The technology for CoolSculpting was developed after a phenomenon called popsicle panniculitis, which was observed in children who sucked on popsicles on one side of their mouth for long periods of time and would end up with an indentation in their cheek because the cold of the popsicle had killed off fat cells. A team of scientists at Harvard took the science of popsicle panniculitis and developed a technology called cryolipolysis, which is marketed under the name CoolSculpting.

CoolSculpting uses a specially designed applicator to freeze the fat cells without damaging the surface of the skin, causing apoptosis (cell death). This allows the body to naturally excrete these damaged fat cells through the liver, resulting in a 20 to 25 percent reduction of the fat layer in the treatment area.

Liposonix

Liposonix® uses high-intensity focused ultrasound (HIFU) to heat and destroy fat cells without damaging the surface of the skin. Similar to CoolSculpting, the body flushes out the damaged cells via the liver, for a permanent reduction of fat in the treated area. Results may be subtle and can take up to three months to see the full results. Pain medication may be required to tolerate the heat and prickly sensation of a Liposonix treatment.

SculpSure

SculpSure® uses targeted laser energy to heat fat cells under the skin. The SculpSure device utilizes cooling throughout the treatment while the laser cycles on and off raising the temperature of the fat cells, damaging their structural integrity. Treatment is well tolerated, with most patients feeling a deep warmth or tingling sensation. Over the next three months, the damaged fat cells are processed and eliminated by the body's lymphatic system. Treated fat cells eliminated during a SculpSure treatment will not regenerate.

TruSculpt

The TruSculpt® device features six small handpieces that can be customized in their placements depending on the patient. TruSculpt pulses monopolar radio-frequency energy below the skin's surface to selectively heat and damage fat cells, which are then excreted from the body. Results are gradual with full results seen at three months.

UltraShape

UltraShape® uses focused, pulsed ultrasound energy to selectively destroy the walls of the fat cells in the treatment area. These fat cells are released from the body in the form of triglycerides and processed and eliminated through the liver. Results may be seen as early as two weeks, and multiple treatments may be required.

Kybella

Kybella® is an injectable treatment of deoxycholic acid, the same type of acid that breaks down dietary fats in the stomach. When injected into the fat beneath the chin, Kybella incites an inflammatory response that permanently destroys the fat cells so they can no longer store or accumulate fat. Multiple injections are required to treat a small area, and patients may experience swelling in the treated area for several days after treatment. Depending on the patient, multiple treatments may be required.

When I personally qualify a patient for noninvasive treatments (a variety of which I offer in my practice), a good candidate is a patient who has smaller areas that need to be reduced and who is not interested in doing surgery, because in the hands of the right surgeon, liposuction surgery will always give a consistently better result than any noninvasive device. But, for a patient who absolutely does not want surgery, noninvasive body contouring procedures are reasonable.

A good candidate for noninvasive contouring should have small, localized areas of fat, such as on the flanks, upper outer or inner thighs, central abdomen, or upper arms. When larger surface areas need to be contoured completely, many times circumferentially, a noninvasive approach doesn't make sense.

Most of the noninvasive technologies currently on the market are not good for skin tightening or skin retraction, which is much more effective with well-done liposuction, particularly with a lot of the newer technologies, such as Renuvion® or BodyTite®.

I have seen numerous patients who have not been evaluated correctly and have undergone noninvasive body contouring that has brought areas of fat down but created disproportion by storing more fat in other untreated areas. This again leads to the importance of the patient evaluation. With certain technologies, such as CoolSculpting, there is a potential for drop-offs, "shelves," or "ledges" if the applicator has been improperly applied. In up to 2 percent of CoolSculpting patients, there can be a paradoxical hypertrophy of fat, where there is an increase of fat in the treatment area.

I have seen several patients in my practice who almost look like revision patients with uneven fat loss, scarring, and pullback of the skin after noninvasive body contouring treatments. This may be due to the improper application of devices, or because the patient was not an ideal candidate for nonsurgical body contouring. They have numerous irregularities and I approach their treatments just like I would for a revision patient.

However, nonsurgical body contouring procedures are here to stay, and I expect them to only grow in popularity in the years ahead. It is up to the provider to use them responsibly, and it is up to the patient to understand if it is truly the right procedure for them.

SECTION 2:
REVISION LIPOSUCTION

INTRODUCTION

Revision liposuction surgery is performed to correct irregularities caused by the previous work of another surgeon. Statistically, liposuction revision surgery is one of the most common revision procedures of any type of cosmetic surgery performed in the United States today.

Liposuction is often not given the respect that it should by the surgeon. It is a difficult surgery to perform well, with many complexities which can lead to high levels of patient dissatisfaction after liposuction surgery. In my experience as a revision liposuction surgeon, I have seen firsthand several common factors that will lead a patient to seek a revision surgery:

1. The surgeon is a jack-of-all-trades, but master of none.

A surgeon may excel at other cosmetic procedures such as rhinoplasties, face-lifts, breast surgeries, and even tummy tucks, but may not have the technical skills needed for liposuction.

2. Liposuction is not given the same degree of priority and respect as other cosmetic surgeries.

Many surgeons view liposuction as just "sucking out the fat," but there is so much more to a great surgical outcome with liposuction.

3. The surgeon does not enjoy performing liposuction as much as other surgeries.

The surgeon may not get into the nuances of the art of liposuction surgery and may view it as simply grunt work. It is a physically and technically demanding surgery that many surgeons, especially as they age, find to be hard on their bodies.

4. Liposuction was performed primarily as a fat-harvesting procedure.

Fat transfer has become an increasingly popular element of many cosmetic surgeries, including Brazilian butt lifts, breast augmentations, and facial contouring procedures. The fat is removed with liposuction from a donor area and is then injected into other areas of the body to create or restore lost volume. Again, this may fall back on the surgeon if they are lacking the skills to do liposuction well. A large part of my revision work is correcting bad liposuction surgeries in donor areas that were treated for fat transfer.

In this section, I will further delve into the factors that lead a patient to seek revision liposuction surgery and how to make informed choices to find the right surgeon.

EMOTIONAL TRUST OF THE PATIENT FOR REVISION WORK

Trusting your surgeon is an important factor for any surgery. Many of my revision patients had trusted their initial surgeon, believing they would be taken to the "promised land" of a great result. When liposuction surgery leads to a poor result, that trust has been broken, leading to emotional trauma. A patient may have been dealing with certain body image issues prior to surgery, and now those issues have been compounded even further.

Any patient who has had cosmetic surgery of any type and has had a less than ideal result is almost always emotionally traumatized from it. Prior to surgery, the patient had put their trust in that surgeon, envisioning a certain result or outcome, and often these decisions are made too quickly.

Price-driven motivations, recommendations from a friend, aggressive marketing tactics, or falling prey to seeking a specific technology instead of doing one's due diligence can lead to a poor outcome. I recommend researching carefully to align yourself with the right surgeon for the best chance of a good result without complications.

When I see patients for revision, they have usually done a lot of research to choose their next surgeon to put their trust in, and they are much less trusting now than they had been before their initial surgery. They have a lot more concerns and questions before going ahead with revision surgery.

This leads to the importance of proper evaluation and technique by the surgeon. I am very sensitive when seeing revision patients and I take care to appreciate what they have been through. Perhaps they no longer trust their initial liposuction surgeon to fix their poor result. In many instances, this may be a wise decision because if the surgeon didn't have the skill set to give them a good result, or if they have caused a bad irregularity, there is a high chance of those issues occurring again.

Many patients have significant trauma associated with their poor results. A high percentage of revision patients will break down and cry during their consultation. There may be guilt that they went through the procedure in the first place. Many were happier with their bodies prior to going through that first surgery, and they now avoid exposing those areas in short skirts or bathing suits because the result can look so unnatural. There may be shame associated with the money they had spent on their poor result, which is compounded further by potentially having to spend more money to have the revision work done.

I have coined the term "sweet, trusting patient syndrome" to describe patients who were sweet and trusting of their surgeon and now don't feel comfortable telling their initial surgeon that they are unhappy with their outcome.

Many surgeons possess a superiority complex and can come across as being overly confident. But patients should always proceed with caution when choosing a surgeon, as one of the most dangerous combinations is a surgeon who has a great bedside manner but lacks the technical skills that lead to a good result.

In my opinion, it is better to have a surgeon who doesn't have a great bedside manner, perhaps they are a little cold or quiet, but they do technically great work. Of course, the best combination is a surgeon who has both—they are warm and have excellent judgment and technical skills.

COMPLEXITY OF REVISION WORK

Any surgeon who performs revision work will say it is by far more complicated than performing the original surgery. This rings true for revision rhinoplasty, revision face-lift surgery, revision breast surgery, and of course, revision liposuction. It is always easier to get the most perfect result the first time.

Revision liposuction surgery is much more complex, which many patients do not understand. For many reasons, it typically is more difficult to go back in the second time, and it may be a more involved process requiring other technologies to make improvements to the poor initial result.

Many surgeons will decline to take on revision liposuction patients because they lack the skills and technical ability to perform it well. It is important with revision liposuction for the surgeon to truly understand what has gone wrong and why a problem has occurred, whether it be a drop-off or shelf-like appearance, or an unnatural shape. Perhaps the irregularity had been caused by the wrong tools being used, or because the surgeon was overly aggressive and didn't appreciate the skin laxity.

Another important factor to revision liposuction is that the surgeon is dealing with tissue that has been made unnatural. The first surgery may have created scar tissue that will now need to be released in a certain way to improve the appearance of indentations and irregularities. This involves a high level of complexity, and the reality is that it may not be possible to make it as perfect as it could have been made the first time around.

CATEGORIES OF PROBLEMS ENCOUNTERED IN REVISION LIPOSUCTION

1. Creating disproportion
2. Disrespecting the "cosmetic unit"
3. Asymmetry
4. Overly conservative
5. Overly aggressive
6. Improper blending
7. Buttock drop
8. Skin irregularities
9. Improper placement of incision points

1. Disproportion and Balance of the Body

The ultimate goal of liposuction surgery is to create overall harmony and balance to a person's body by targeting disproportionate areas. These are areas that genetically store fat unevenly. When a person gains fat, it tends to go to those disproportionate areas first, and when weight is lost, it comes off those areas less. The main role of liposuction is to fix those areas of disproportion. A surgeon can run the risk of creating disproportion if they do not look at the proportions of the entire body.

A common scenario in cosmetic surgery is a patient who may be around thirty pounds overweight but not disproportionate. They may be seeing a surgeon for another procedure, like breast implants or rhinoplasty, and in the consultation they ask about the excess weight they are carrying around their abdomen. The surgeon asks to take a look, the patient lifts their shirt and shows the fullness in that area, and the surgeon says, "Sure. Let's do liposuction to get rid of that for you." And they add it to the estimate. The mistake this surgeon has made is that they didn't look at the entire body from the neck down to the feet, from a standpoint of overall harmony and balance. The patient may in fact be proportionate in their weight gain over their entire body, and not just in their abdomen. When the surgeon performs liposuction only to the abdomen, that patient will start storing fat unevenly in other areas of their body, creating disproportion. Correcting disproportion created from previous liposuction surgery is a big part of the revision work I perform.

2. Disproportion and Balance of the "Cosmetic Unit"

Disproportion and balance of the "cosmetic unit" (as discussed in a previous chapter) is another very important concept for revision liposuction. The body should be looked at not only for overall harmony and balance, but also for the harmony and balance of each individual "cosmetic unit".

For example, liposuction to the lower abdomen is a fairly common procedure. The surgeon should look at the entire "cosmetic unit", which may include fullness in the upper abdomen and waistline. When the entire "cosmetic unit" is not addressed, untreated areas (such as the upper back) can start to store fat disproportionately within that "cosmetic unit", creating an unnatural "bat wing"

1. Address the body in "cosmetic units". Additional liposuction may be required to achieve "balance and proportion".

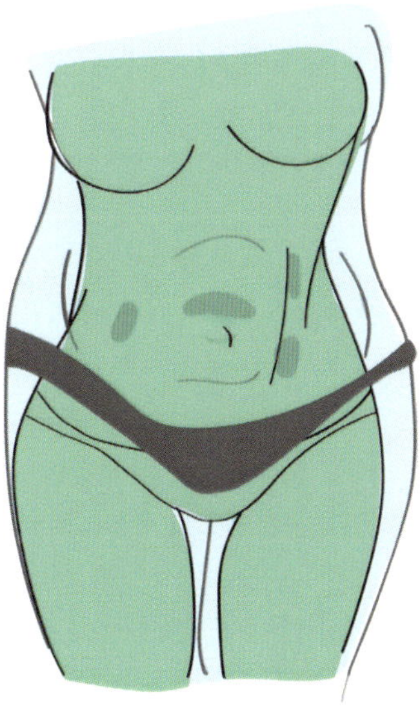

2. Gentle liposuction may be needed to smooth out areas to help lift skin.

3. Fat grafting may be required in areas that were over liposuctioned.

4. Due to stretched skin and trauma to connective tissue, J-Plasma may be used to tighten loose skin, or in cases of severe skin laxity, a tummy tuck may be recommended.

appearance. Another consideration is that the skin of the untreated upper back will not have contracted, and it may hang over the contracted areas below, which will worsen as time goes on.

This can also occur with the thigh area. A patient may have had liposuction to their outer thighs only, but in respect to the "cosmetic unit", they should have had both their outer and inner thighs treated to create the right type of three-dimensional balance. A patient who has fat that wraps around the entire thigh area may have Lipedema, which should be approached in a circumferential manner to balance the entire "cosmetic unit".

3. Asymmetry

Asymmetry can often be fairly easy to fix. Generally, the human body is symmetrical. Some patients may have more muscle bulk, a slightly different bone shape, or a tilt of the pelvis, creating more fullness on one side than the other. In these cases, a surgeon may perform overly aggressive liposuction on one side, creating asymmetry. The body then needs to be rebalanced and made more symmetrical.

A patient may say their right hip or thigh is larger than their left. In my experience, it's almost always due to an underlying skeletal issue where one leg may be longer than the other, sometimes by as much as an inch. This will cause the pelvis to tilt to one side. This will be visible often in the crease on the buttock, where one crease is slightly higher than the other.

It is important for a patient to understand that some asymmetry may exist in their body prior to liposuction surgery that may not be able to be completely corrected. It may be possible to "cheat" a little bit by bringing the fuller side down a bit more with liposuction, but you may not be able to completely correct that natural asymmetry.

4. Incomplete or Overly Conservative Treatment

Revision of incomplete or overly conservative liposuction is probably the easiest category to correct. If a surgeon has a choice of being too aggressive or too conservative, it really is better to treat the patient conservatively because it is easier to make corrections in a subsequent revision procedure.

5. Overly Aggressive Treatment

More often than not, the patient wants the surgeon to remove every single bit of fat. This aggressive approach can lead to disaster. I see many patients from surgeons in my area who have a reputation for being too aggressive, leading to a lot of problems. A surgeon should always temper how aggressive they are being in each patient, based on a number of factors.

One factor is the elasticity and thickness of the skin. In certain areas where there is good skin elasticity or thickness (such as the back), a surgeon can be more aggressive and complete without causing skin irregularities. Other areas (like the inner thighs or abdomen of women in their fifties and sixties with delicate, thin skin, almost like the skin of the eyelid) should be approached with caution to prevent uneven pullback of the skin.

A condition called erythema ab liporaspiration (coined by Dr. Jeffrey Klein, who developed the tumescent liposuction technique) can occur when the surgeon has been too aggressive. The skin takes on a mottled purplish-red and white lace-like pattern, almost like looking through very thin skin to the underlying vasculature. This can be almost impossible to correct and will likely be permanent and unresponsive to revision liposuction or laser treatments.

6. Improper Blending and Unnatural Shape

It is common to see improper blending or an unnatural shape in revision liposuction patients. This occurs when the entire "cosmetic unit" is not respected, leaving drop-offs or "shelves" caused by improper blending. The surgeon should always blend the area they are treating into the surrounding tissue to create a gradual, smooth transition. Revision of a drop-off or "shelf" may involve further liposuction to blend and smooth into the surrounding area, or a fat transfer may be required to soften the transition.

Another aspect of improper blending is an unnatural shape. This is common in the outer thigh "saddlebag" area where the surgeon can create an unnatural shape by being overly aggressive. Many times, that surgeon has tried to create a more contoured shape to the buttocks and outer thigh areas and has tried to accentuate the natural buttock crease, leading to an unnatural shape and the telltale sign that the patient has had liposuction surgery. The patient's curves may now take on a masculine, straight up and down appearance, or the buttock takes on an inverted appearance where they are wider in the hips and flanks and narrower in their outer buttocks area.

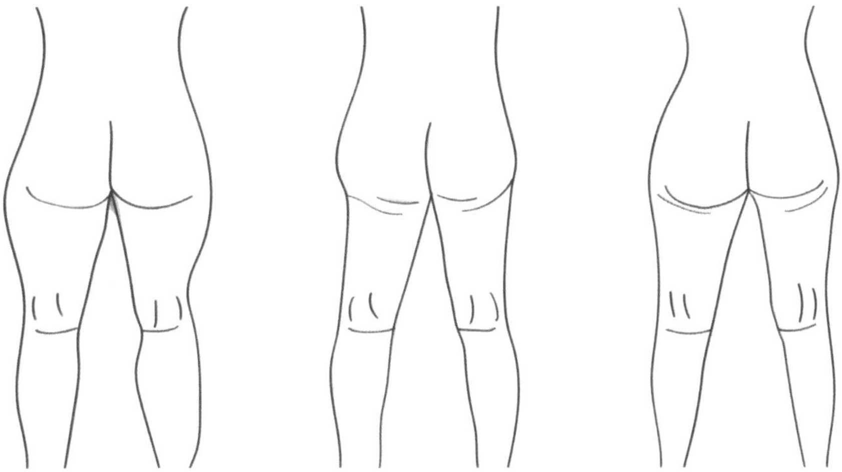

Before liposuction

After overly aggressive liposuction. Note the loss of natural curves.

After revision liposuction and fat grafting

When liposuction is performed on the lower abdomen only, without proper blending into the upper abdomen, it can lead to an unnatural retraction where the upper abdomen can hang down and cause the belly button to take on the appearance of a downturned frown.

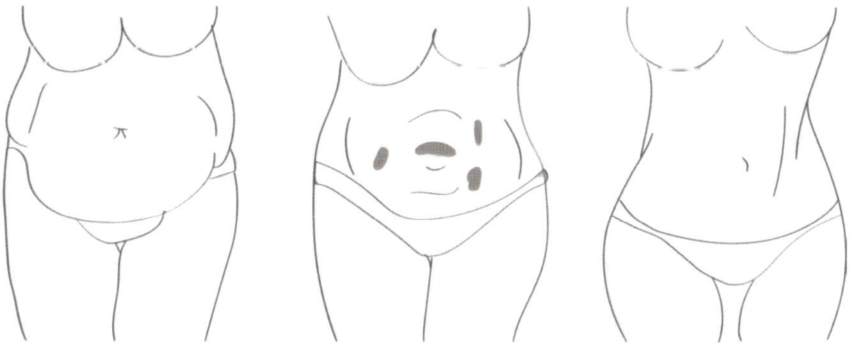

Before liposuction

After botched liposuction

After revision liposuction and fat grafting

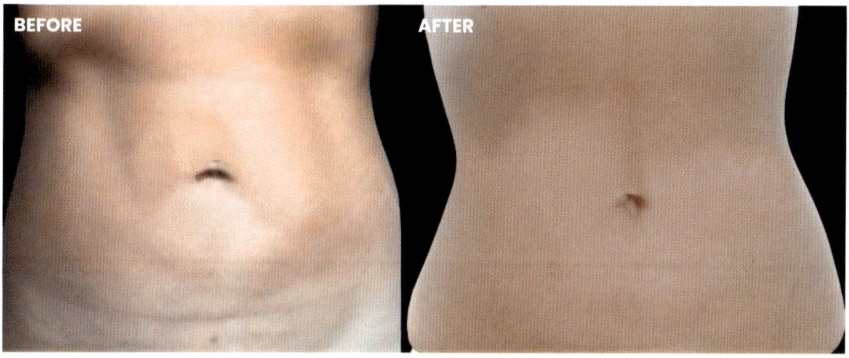

Above: Before and after revision liposuction to the abdomen

For best results, liposuction should always be approached in a three-dimensional, circumferential manner to prevent the body from taking on an unnatural shape. Incision points and positioning are important factors, as many of the tools used in liposuction surgery are straight and do not follow the natural curvature of the body.

7. Buttock Drop

A buttock drop is an unfortunate occurrence that can be caused by overly aggressive liposuction to the lower buttock "banana roll" area. Going too deeply in this area can cause the fibrous support tissues that support the buttocks to release, and one buttock will drop in relation to the other. In these cases, the issue may be difficult or impossible to correct.

8. Skin Irregularities

Skin irregularities are probably the most common complication people think of with bad liposuction surgery, and it is unfortunately very common. Virtually every revision patient I've seen has had some degree of skin irregularities. This occurs primarily because of disrespect for the skin, and it leads back to the importance of staying within the "safe plane" (discussed in Section 1: Cosmetic Liposuction) when performing liposuction surgery.

When performing liposuction, most surgeons don't pay much attention to the skin and will often disrespect it by jabbing, poking, and dragging the cannula, or by simply being too aggressive. They may jab the skin from underneath with the tip of a cannula, or drag the cannula underneath the skin, creating obvious cannula marks. If energy-based devices are being used, there is a risk of burning or heating the skin from underneath, and the skin may respond by forming uneven scar tissue.

When liposuction is performed correctly, an even sheet of connective scar tissue will retract the skin evenly. If it is performed improperly with any disrespect, the skin will respond by retracting unevenly, causing an irregularity I call tethering. This is where the scarring under the skin can pull back unevenly, and the skin can now be attached to the muscle underneath—and that looser skin on the top can settle in relation to that tethered skin and create more irregularities.

Tethering can commonly be seen in the abdomen, thighs, and knees. It is less common in areas with thicker skin, such as the back, or in the taut skin of the calves and ankles. This leads back to the importance of properly supporting the skin during surgery. If a surgical technician is torquing or twisting the skin while the surgeon is performing liposuction underneath, it could cause an irregularity of the skin when it settles down. I've seen many surgeons grab the skin and almost pinch it up with their hands and liposuction aggressively underneath. This is a poor technique that will just create irregularities to the skin.

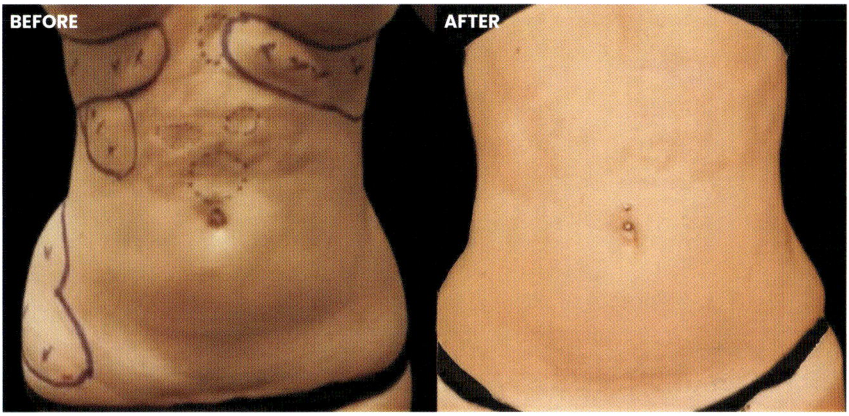

Above: This patient presented with obvious skin irregularities post liposuction. The image on the right shows her result after revision liposuction.

Pearl for the Surgeon

Make sure the skin is always stretched as a tight sheet when liposuctioning areas of looser skin. Make sure there is always proper counter-retraction with your free hand, as well as with the hands of the surgical technician.

9. Incision Points

The improper placement of incision points can absolutely affect the outcome of liposuction surgery. Liposuction should generally be performed along the axis of natural skin tension lines, generally in a vertical direction for most areas of the body.

Going in a horizontal direction—particularly if the surgeon is not respectful of the skin, and if the cannula is dragged underneath—can create a rippled type of irregularity. An example of this can be seen in the outer thigh area. If the surgeon is using an incision point underneath the buttock and is going around the outer thigh area horizontally and disrespecting the skin, when it settles, the irregularity will take place in a rippled fashion. Approaching this area vertically typically leads to a smoother result.

While the upper back is an area not usually prone to irregularities, if the surgeon is using incision points around the spine and trying to go around the rib cage in a horizontal direction on the skin (instead of approaching vertically), the skin will catch and be tethered, taking on a rippled appearance.

Thin, delicate skin should always be respected as it is more prone to irregularities. The surgeon should approach liposuction conservatively in areas of reduced elasticity. The greater thickness and skin tautness in an area, the less prone it is to irregularity.

As a person ages, their skin loses elasticity. When performing liposuction on a twenty-year-old male, the skin will be quite taut and will retract evenly, so it can be approached more aggressively. Whereas a woman in her forties who has had three children will have a certain degree of looseness and loss of elasticity to her abdomen area and should be treated conservatively with caution.

The most important factor for incision points is where they are strategically placed. Once an area is defined to be liposuctioned, sculpting should always be approached by an incision point strategically placed at the perimeter of the defined field—almost never within the field. In much of my revision work, I see improper placement of an incision point as one of the main causes of a poor result.

Pearl for the Surgeon

Always approach liposuction of an area from the perimeter, preferably respecting natural skin tension lines.

STRATEGIES AND TECHNIQUES

As a revision surgeon, I strongly feel that it's important for the patient to understand the exact strategy the surgeon is suggesting for their revision surgery. The patient should really try to pin down their revision surgeon to their exact strategy to correct the problem and make sure that the surgeon has evaluated the complete body.

When I see a patient for revision liposuction surgery, I analyze their entire body so I can understand what has caused the problem. I don't rely on simply asking the patient; I can see what has been improperly blended, or where the previous surgeon has been too aggressive. This gives me insight into what has caused the problem and I can then find the starting point to determine what is needed to make improvements.

When I see a patient for a revision liposuction consultation, 90 to 95 percent of the time I can help them with revision work. It's important for the surgeon to have really good judgment about when revision liposuction is viable for further improvement, or when a revision surgery may make things worse. This applies to all types of revision cosmetic surgeries.

I have three questions that I discuss with patients regarding areas of improvement:

1. What is my assessment of the percentage chance that I'm going to be able to make the flaws significantly better?

I am specifically using the phrase "significantly better." I do not use the terms "gone," "complete," or "perfect" because it may be impossible to make things completely perfect, but I want to be able to make it significantly better so the patient can come away from their surgery feeling like it was worthwhile. For simplicity, let's say that the degree of improvement is greater than 50 percent.

2. What is the percentage chance that improvement may be slight or insignificant?

Perhaps after revision surgery there has not been as much improvement as the surgeon and patient had wanted, and there was an improvement of around 30 percent.

To me, significant improvement would be above 50 percent, ideally 70, 80, or even 90 percent better. I would say an insignificant improvement would be around 20 to 30 percent improvement. Some patients may not have any improvements at all. This was of course not the goal, but it's important to note that the result is not ultimately worse.

3. What is the percentage chance that revision surgery will make things worse?

This should be an extremely small number, 1 percent or less. For me, it starts at around a 5 percent chance that I feel revision surgery should not be performed due to the risk of making things worse. Patients are typically investing their hope and money into it, so I feel that is important for the surgeon to be realistic with the patient regarding expectations about the outcome of a revision surgery. I pride myself in that, although I may not always meet a patient's expectations, I have never created worse problems in a revision patient.

STRATEGIES TO CORRECT PROBLEMS IN REVISION LIPOSUCTION SURGERY

For the vast majority of revision patients, they typically have several problems that need to be addressed. There may be disproportion, unnatural shapes, and skin irregularities often represented in one patient. Below are several categories for the different strategies I will apply to various problems that can occur with liposuction:

Rebalancing of Disproportion

Fixing disproportion often comes down to rebalancing the entire body. It's looking from the standpoint of where the disproportion is occurring on a patient who possibly should have never had liposuction in the first place. I often ask my patients if they had areas of stubborn or disproportionate fat prior to their initial liposuction surgery. Many times, the answer is no. The patient was in proportion in their teenage years and twenties, so that surgeon has made that patient disproportioned. The entire body should be considered from the neck down to determine where the disproportion is and how to go about correcting it. It may mean a number of areas will require treatment.

Rebalancing the "Cosmetic Unit"

If the "cosmetic unit" was treated partially, the untreated areas may need to be addressed to rebalance the entire "cosmetic unit" as a whole. One of the most common examples I see in my practice is the partial treatment of the torso, where the middle and upper parts of the back did not receive treatment. Going in and rebalancing this untreated area allows the skin to retract evenly so it becomes harmonious with the rest of the torso "cosmetic unit".

In revision liposuction, if the previous surgeon has made the patient disproportionate, the "cosmetic unit" may require circumferential treatment, particularly in Lipedema patients. If just the inner and outer thighs have been treated without the surgeon realizing the patient had Lipedema, revision liposuction of the entire "cosmetic unit" may be required to restore the optimal shape to that unit.

Correcting Asymmetry

To use the thighs as an example, a patient who had one thigh treated more aggressively than the other, leading to asymmetry, may require the other thigh to be brought down further. Or, depending on the deformity, a fat transfer may be required to correct the asymmetry and create a more natural appearance and silhouette.

Correcting an Incomplete or Overly Conservative Treatment

This is typically one of the easiest concerns to correct. If an area was not treated enough, there is a potential for the skin to retract unevenly. Going back in and treating these unaddressed areas may allow for skin tightening on the areas that have gravitationally settled and will allow those areas to retract more completely. Many times, I will add skin-tightening techniques with energy-based devices such as Renuvion® or radio-frequency BodyTite® to obtain greater skin tightening.

Correcting an Overly Aggressive Treatment

Correcting an overly aggressive treatment can be very challenging, particularly in areas where the skin could not support aggressive treatment. A common area where this may occur is the abdomen. A variety of techniques may need to be employed to release the scar tissue and make improvements.

I typically use a multistep process in my practice that begins with hydrodissecting and releasing the scar tissue with tumescent fluid. I then go back in with what I call vibrosection, which is the mechanical release of scar tissue with a power-assisted liposuction device with the suction itself turned off and the use of specific dissecting cannulas. This is followed by VASER, which is ultrasonic energy to emulsify the fat layer and then coat the skin with an oily substance, allowing it to pull back in a more even fashion.

Depending on the patient I may include a skin-tightening device such as Renuvion or BodyTite to areas of tethering to allow that skin to retract more evenly. Finally, a fat transfer may be required to build up an area with an unnatural shape.

Correcting Skin Irregularities

For correcting skin irregularities, I typically take a step-by-step approach that begins with hydrodissection with fluid, vibrosection with mechanical release, VASER emulsification to coat the skin with oil, skin tightening, and then possible fat transfer to the area.

Patients who are being treated for skin irregularities will benefit from the proper use of compression after revision surgery. In my practice I will often use compression foams such as Epifoam®or Reston™ to achieve even retraction of the skin underneath the compression garment that the patient will wear for typically up to several weeks. This gives the skin the greatest chance of pulling back in an even fashion.

SECTION 3: LIPEDEMA

WHAT IS LIPEDEMA?

Lipedema is a disproportionate fat storage disease that is extremely underrecognized not only in the United States but around the world. It was identified in a 1940 landmark paper by Drs. Allen and Hines of the Mayo Clinic in Rochester, Minnesota,[vi] and in a subsequent paper in 1947 by the same authors.[vii] However, Lipedema is widely ignored within the medical community and the condition is not on the syllabus in medical schools.

As a result, patients are often misdiagnosed with obesity, lymphedema, or elephantiasis. Personally, I feel the name Lipedema is confusing and too similar in name to lymphedema, which is a buildup of lymph fluid. I have suggested that the medical community change the name Lipedema to Lipofibroedema as it is more accurate and sounds like a significant condition.

Lipedema largely affects women, with up to 11 percent of the female population—approximately 17 million American women and 370 million women worldwide—affected with varying degrees of Lipedema.

Lipedema is a misunderstood disease that typically presents in puberty. There is definitely a genetic component to Lipedema, and the condition increases in severity throughout a person's lifetime. It is usually an insidious process, but it may increase with pregnancy, menopause, OB-GYN surgery, or hormonal changes.

Patients as young as nine years old may start to show subtle signs of Lipedema, which is why I am so passionate about educating the public and the medical community—specifically pediatricians and OB-GYNs—to diagnose the disease when it starts presenting around puberty.

There are many misunderstandings and a great lack of awareness around Lipedema. There is pervasive ignorance with regard to the disease, and while ignorance doesn't necessarily indicate stupidity, it does mean that the condition has been ignored for way too long. It's unfortunate that it is still so underrecognized by the medical community and insurance companies, as it becomes a real hardship for patients. Hopefully this will change in the near future.

LIPEDEMA DIAGNOSIS

The diagnosis of Lipedema is extremely important and should ideally be determined at the earliest age possible—even at or around puberty—so as much can be done as possible to slow the progression of the disease.

The name itself, Lipedema, is not really inaccurate: it is a combination of fat and swelling. However, there is another component that I would like to see represented in the name, which is the fibrous element that causes scar tissue and inflammation, so I have suggested the term Lipofibroedema.

Lipedema presents in puberty and is most certainly a genetically inherited condition that appears to follow an autosomal dominant inheritance pattern, passing down from generation to generation. Lipedema can be inherited directly from the mother or father in equal frequency, so when looking at family history, it's not only important to look at the mother's side but also the women on the father's side of the family.

Around half of the time, with autosomal dominant inheritance patterns, the disease is picked up from the father. And in some patients, because it is such a common condition, the gene may be picked up from both sides of the family. Men carry the gene as frequently as women do, but the disease is very rarely expressed in men while it is commonly expressed in women. There is a 50 percent chance that a person who has Lipedema or is carrying the gene will pass it down to an offspring.

The diagnosis of Lipedema is dependent on the signs, characteristics, and symptoms of the disease. In medical terminology, signs refers to the appearance of how the Lipedema presents, and the symptoms include pain and discomfort.

Diagnosis of Lipedema

Signs

- Column-like appearance of the legs and/or arms
- Fullness in the upper buttocks
- Fullness in the upper arms and possibly also in the forearms

Symptoms

- Pain
- Swelling
- Easy bruising
- Hypermobile joints and/or skin

Family History

- On either maternal or paternal side

The Signs, Stages, and Types of Lipedema

There are different stages of severity of Lipedema that range from stage 1 to stage 4 (Lipolymphedema), with stage 1 being the mildest and stage 4 being the most advanced. Symptoms of pain may not always be related to severity of stage. There are also several distinct patterns of distribution known as "types."

An important differentiator between a patient with Lipedema and a person with genetically fat thighs is the pattern of distribution. In my practice I do a lot of virtual consultations where I'm looking at photographs of a patient, and I can diagnose Lipedema almost immediately based on the pattern of distribution that the Lipedema exhibits, forming a circumferential column-like appearance. A patient with fat thighs typically has fat in the inner or outer thigh areas, whereas in someone with Lipedema that fat encircles the entire leg. There is commonly as much fullness in the anterior and posterior component of the leg as there is in the outer and inner thighs.

There is another slightly less common pattern of Lipedema which involves primarily the hips, upper buttocks (pelvic girdle), and circumferential thights down to the knees. In this pattern the calves and ankles are either spared or have minimal involvement.

In my extensive experience of liposuction to the calves and ankles, patients with fat calves and ankles who do not have Lipedema will typically have fat in the posterior two-thirds of the calf and ankle units. Lipedema of the calves and ankles obliterates the tibia (shin-bone), and you start to lose definition and shape to the lower leg as it is a circumferential process.

Similarly, in the upper arms, many women have fat that begins to cause the backs of the arms to drop as they age, but with Lipedema the differentiator it is that the fat and swelling has wrapped around the whole upper arm—even on the top part of the arm—and again, the arm starts to lose definition and shape.

Another important clue is the characteristic appearance of a Lipedema patient. Many of these patients are extremely disproportionate. They tend to have very little fullness in their torso area but are very disproportionate in their extremities (their entire leg and arm units).

Stages of Lipedema

Stage 1 - Mild circumferential fullness with skin that is soft and smooth.

Stage 2 - Moderate circumferential fullness with development of irregularities of skin surface and subcutaneous nodules.

Stage 3 - Advanced circumferential fullness typically with development of lobules and increasing hardening of tissue due to fibrosis.

Stage 4 - Very advanced circumferential fullness with large overhanging masses of tissues with prominent hardening due to damage of lymphatic vessels resulting in secondary Lymphedema (Lipolymphedema).

Types of Lipedema

Type I - Fat localized to upper buttocks, hips, and lower abdomen (pelvic girdle).

Type II - Fat involving pelvic girdle down the thighs circumferentially to the knees.

Type III - Fat involves pelvis down to ankles circumferentially (most common pattern).

Type IV - Fat involves upper arms circumferentially and potential involvement of forearms down to the wrist.

Type V - Fat involves calves circumferentially from knees to ankles.

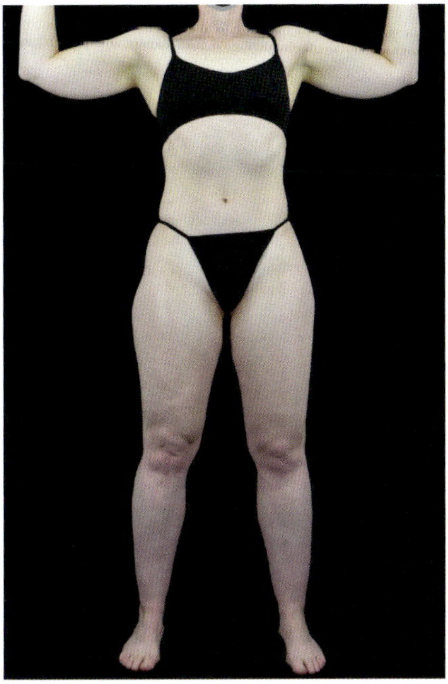

Above: Lipedema Stage 1

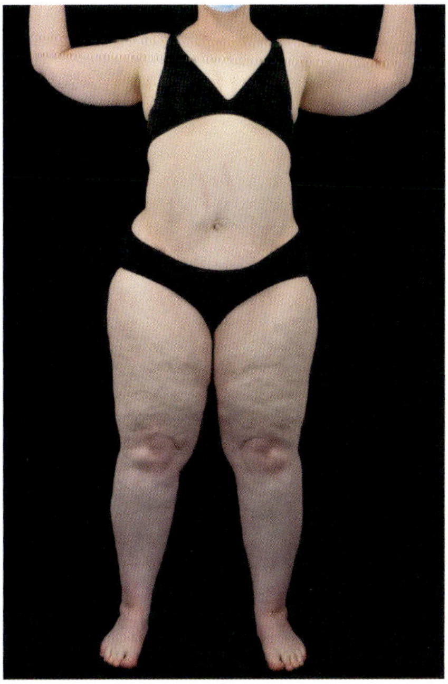

Above: Lipedema Stage 2

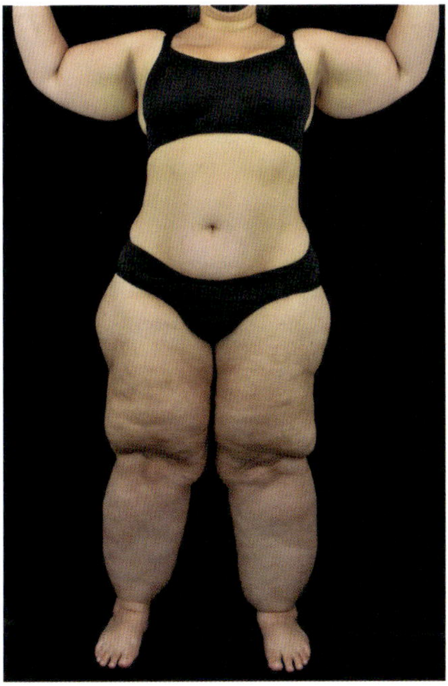

Above: Lipedema Stage 3

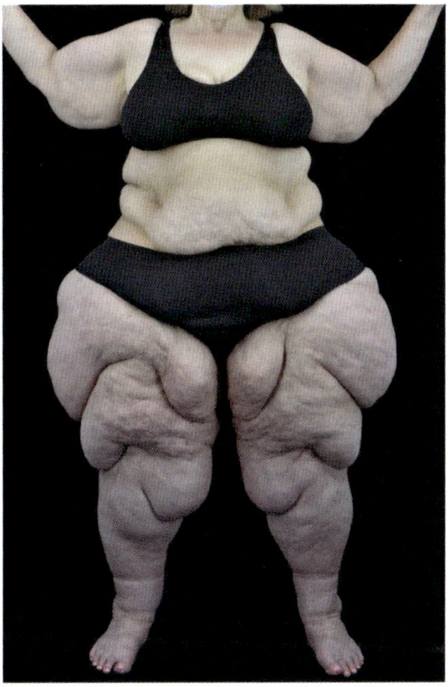

Above: Lipedema Stage 4

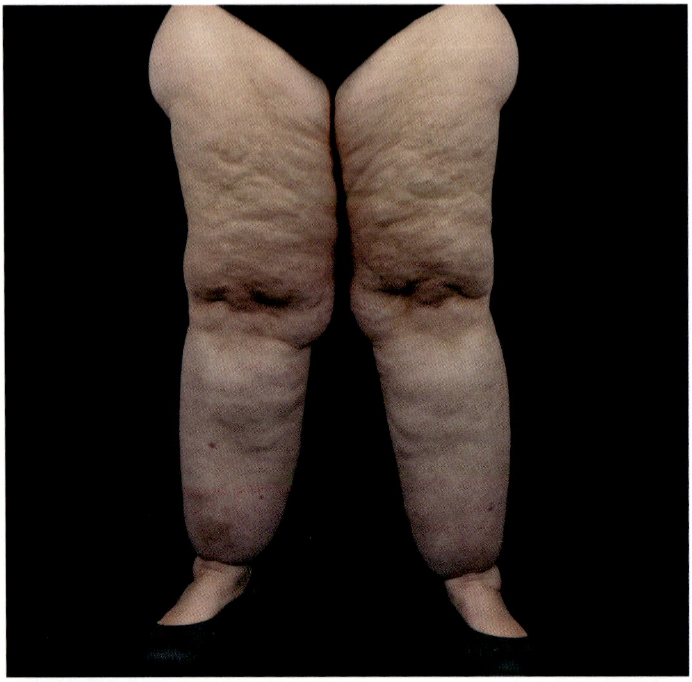

Above: Type III column-like pattern

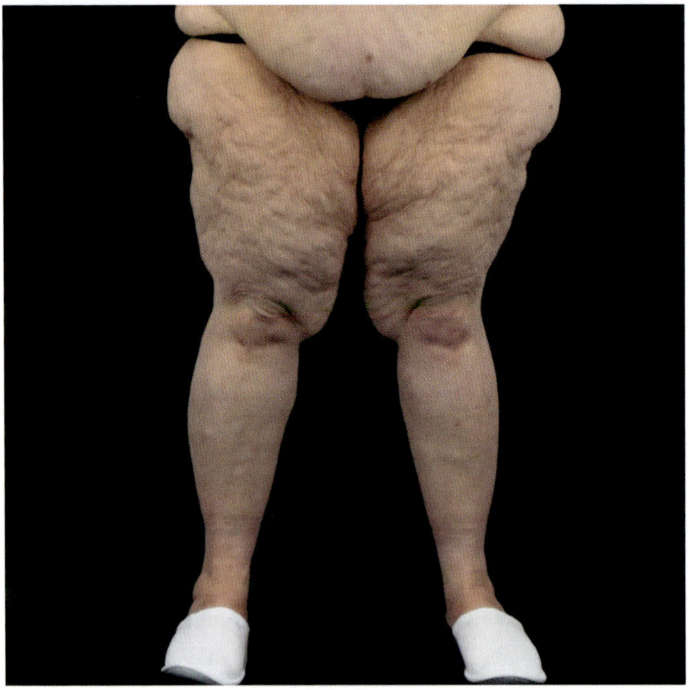

Above: Type II triangular-like pattern

The Symptoms of Lipedema

Pain

Pain is a characteristic symptom of Lipedema, and it can be extremely variable and is not always dependent on the stage of Lipedema. For example, a stage 4 patient may be quite large and yet have almost no pain, while a stage 1 patient may be in excruciating pain. This has a lot to do with how much inflammation is present, which in turn affects how much fibrosis is in the affected areas. The pain typically follows a characteristic pattern, and it commonly presents as pain and sensitivity to pressure. For example, a Lipedema patient may have a lot of pain from the pressure of a massage, or they may have a lot more sensitivity when someone puts their hand on their leg or when their pet jumps across their thighs. In either case, it's typically a pain to pressure. Many patients think their pain is normal and they realize after surgery, when the pain goes away, that it wasn't normal.

Lipedema pain may also be described as a dull ache throughout the leg. There may also be some sharp areas of pain that the patient may complain about. Sometimes the pain is consistent throughout the day, or the patient may experience excruciating pain that wakes them up at night.

Swelling

The next characteristic symptom is swelling, which is caused by the movement of fluid across the lymphatic membrane. The degree of swelling can vary from patient to patient. Some are fairly stable with minimal swelling, while others may have significant swelling. For some patients, the swelling may increase or decrease throughout the day with changes in temperature, altitude, or positioning.

Easy Bruising

Another common symptom of Lipedema is how easily a patient will bruise. There is a fragility to the capillary wall that coincides with Lipedema, and the vast majority of Lipedema patients complain of bruising easily.

Hypermobility of Joints

Approximately 80 to 85 percent of Lipedema patients have varying degrees of a condition called Ehlers-Danlos syndrome that goes along with their Lipedema. They have hypermobility of their joints and may be able to bend their thumbs or fingers back easily. Their body can be much more flexible in the hip flexors and such.

Mobile, Loose Skin

Another symptom that goes along with Ehlers-Danlos syndrome is that Lipedema patients have a much more pliable, loose quality to their skin.

Defective Connective Tissue

We know that Lipedema patients have leaky lymphatics, which is caused by a defect in the connective tissue where there is a lack of integrity of the lymphatic walls. Patients with Lipedema may also experience leaky gut syndrome, where fluid moves outside of the intestinal walls causing bloating in the abdominal cavity. Associated symptoms may include brain fog, which is caused by swelling in the central nervous system and brain.

Some patients may even experience impaired proprioception, also referred to as kinesthesia. Proprioception is the medical term that describes the ability to sense the orientation and movement of your body in your environment. When proprioception is impaired, it results in difficulty with basic functional mobility and balance. This is caused by swelling in the peripheral tissues affecting the sensory nerves that are related to the central nervous system. Many Lipedema patients experience balance issues, not just because of their weight but also because of impaired proprioception.

I have predicted for many years that we will find that Lipedema at its core may not simply be a fat disorder. I believe the fat over-growth and swelling are results of a connective tissue disorder which falls into the category of medicine called collagen vascular disorders—such as Ehlers-Danlos syndrome—because there are so many commonalities.

PATHOPHYSIOLOGY

Lipedema is a complicated systemic condition that affects many areas throughout the body. However, it commonly presents itself in the arms, legs, and upper buttocks. Less commonly, the process may involve the abdomen or even the back.

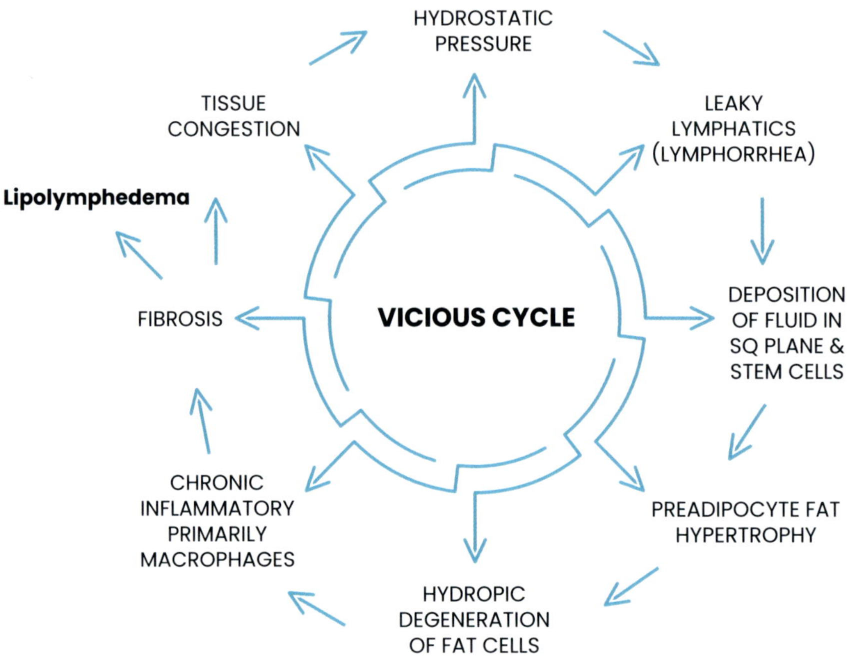

The pathophysiology seems to point to the fact that Lipedema is a combination of fat and swelling in areas caused by a lack of integrity of connective tissue. Research has shown that there is an increased permeability through the walls of the lymphatics where fluid is leaking into the surrounding tissues. Stem cells in the subcutaneous layer of fat become programmed to turn into preadipocytes, which are early fat cells that start replicating very rapidly. Those cells then die off by a process called hydropic degeneration with a turnover so fast that it can't support their survival. One then gets fat cell hypertrophy where the cells are actually duplicating and replicating.

The dying cells then incite inflammation. The inflammation is primarily the result of macrophages that are cleaning up the debris of the dying fat cells, which then incites chronic inflammation and fibrosis (the medical term for scar tissue) within that layer of fat. As the condition progresses, more fibrosis forms, leading to an increase in congestion and hydrostatic pressure within the tissues. This develops into a vicious cycle of more fluid going out due to increased congestion.

In the long term, the fibrotic tissue can begin to permanently damage the lymphatic vessels, resulting in a condition called lipo-lymphedema. This underscores the importance of interrupting the process with surgery and the use of preventative strategies such as compression and specific dietary programs to slow the progression of disease.

THE EMOTIONAL ASPECTS OF LIPEDEMA

Lipedema has a profound emotional impact on almost every patient. In my practice, from the initial consultation to the diagnosis, to weeks, days, or months after surgery, the vast majority of Lipedema patients will cry at some point in their journey because they have been carrying the emotional weight caused by the disease for so long.

Senior Lipedema patients in their sixties and seventies have lived with their condition for decades. Lipedema presents itself at a very sensitive age: adolescence. During the pubertal period or peri-pubertal period, when Lipedema develops, a young girl may be confused about why her body is different from those of her peers, leading to feelings of shame and guilt. She may be made fun of by friends or family members and may be told that she is fat or overweight. Her legs may be pointed out as being "funny-looking." This is then reinforced by the medical community. A doctor may tell the young girl or her parents that she simply needs to diet and exercise more. Fitness professionals may tell her she is not exercising in the right way—yet the fat does not budge.

Many Lipedema patients are constantly looking for what they can do to change their bodies, whether it's cosmetic surgery or weight loss surgery. The lack of control and the inability to improve their symptoms can lead to guilt, shame, frustration, and anger. When they are diagnosed with Lipedema, they are filled with emotions about why they had not been diagnosed earlier so they could have slowed its progression.

In addition to the lack of recognition of Lipedema in the medical community, health insurance companies may not recognize or cover the treatment of Lipedema, leading patients to pay out of pocket for their treatment. This can be incredibly frustrating when other treatment options such as weight loss surgery are routinely covered by insurance companies. But finally and fortunately, health insurance companies are recognizing Lipedema as a disease, and beginning to cover its treatment.

Lipedema patients may develop body dysmorphia, particularly in today's age of social media, where adolescents are being conditioned into thinking they must look a certain way. Patients may lose confidence because they don't know what is happening to their bodies, and they may end up gaining more weight, leading to obesity.

In my practice, I routinely hear how Lipedema has affected my patients' lives. They may be living with significant fear about their future and about their mobility issues. Are they going to be able to walk, or play with their children and grandchildren? There may also be fear of hormonal changes, pregnancy, and menopause worsening their condition.

The emotional impact of Lipedema may also be shared by the patient's entire family. The spouses are almost always loving and supportive. Often it is the spouse who has researched and found the diagnosis and treatment on the internet. When I perform surgeries on these patients, it is such a life-changing experience for the patient that their partners will often hug me!

Years ago, patients didn't know where to go for guidance and information. Thankfully, in the last decade there has been an increase of awareness for Lipedema through the media and internet, but it needs to get better.

WEIGHT LOSS, THE BMI INDEX, AND LIPEDEMA

The vast majority of patients with Lipedema have struggled with their bodies their whole lives and have been told to simply diet and exercise, by family members, friends, and medical professionals. Most go down the "rabbit hole" of weight loss therapies.

Many culminate their journey with weight loss surgery having been misdiagnosed as simply obese based on archaic BMI (body mass index) indexes developed in the early 1800's. Patients with Lipedema undergoing weight loss surgery will almost certainly lose weight, but it is probable that their legs or arms will not change much, and their symptoms will persist. Non-Lipedema fat responds to weight loss, but Lipedema fat rarely does. In my opinion, weight loss surgery should almost never be employed as a treatment for Lipedema. Bariatric surgeons should ideally screen for Lipedema rather than proceeding with patients who qualify for weight loss surgery simply because they are obese based on the BMI index.

There is an exciting new category of medication for weight loss and diabetes, the GLP-1 agonists (Ozempic®, Mounjaro®, Rybelsus® and Wegovy®). This new category of medications is a game changer for weight loss and the management of diabetes. The method of action of this class of medications is primarily to induce weight loss through the reduction of hunger and food intake. However, as important and revolutionary as this new class of medications are, they have a limited role in the treatment of Lipedema. Patients will lose weight but like other weight loss strategies, their Lipedema will generally not significantly improve. This is not only to be expected but is also what I have seen and heard from my Lipedema patients on GLP-1 agonists.

That said, there are anecdotal reports from patients who have experienced a reduction in their inflammation and pain after beginning

GLP-1 agonists. Whether this is due to the reduction of intake of inflammatory foods, or by some other mechanism, remains to be identified. While this improvement of symptoms occurs in the minority of patients trying these medications, the risks, so far, of GLP-1 agonists appear to be minimal. If a Lipedema patient has a positive response, and the medication is well tolerated, it is reasonable to continue the medications prior to surgery.

However, one of my concerns is that patients with more advanced Lipedema may spend time and energy on these medications losing weight but their Lipedema will progress with more fibrosis, possibly resulting in Lipolymphedema. The primary role I see for these medications in Lipedema therapy would primarily be after Lipedema surgery. At this point the Lipedema has been properly treated and the fibrosis decongested. GLP-1 agonists may play a role in additional weight loss of non-Lipedema fat in select patients after recovery from Lipedema surgery.

DIET AND NUTRITION

Common food items can play a role in adversely affecting Lipedema and can speed its progression by increasing the movement of fluid across lymphatic membranes or creating more inflammation. When dietary changes are implemented that are respectful of Lipedema, it can slow its progression—and I use the term "diet" in respect of Lipedema, not simply "dieting."

Inflammatory foods that may need to be avoided to hasten the progression of Lipedema include refined grains, gluten, added sugars, and chemically modified fats. A whole-food, plant-based diet that limits animal products and high-salt foods appears to help with Lipedema.[viii]

Many patients have tried to lose weight to improve their Lipedema symptoms to no avail, because they were dieting in a way that was not respectful of Lipedema. Adhering to a diet strategy that decreases inflammation—such as a low-carbohydrate, ketogenic, or RAD diet—commonly slows the progression of the disease.

Supplements

The use of certain anti-inflammatory dietary supplements may also help to reduce fibrosis, including:

- Vitamin D3
- Vitamin C
- Calcium
- Magnesium
- Omega-3s
- Selenium
- Butcher's Broom
- L-Arginine
- Pycnogenol
- Turmeric
- Alpha-Lipoic Acid
- Bioflavonoids
- Diosmin
- Ashwagandha
- Green Tea
- L-Carnitine
- Chromium
- Dandelion Root
- Quercetin
- MPFF (Micronized Purified Flavonoid Fraction)

COMPRESSION THERAPY

The use of compression therapy in Lipedema is vital and plays an essential role in the treatment of virtually every patient with Lipedema. Combining compression therapy with a respectful dietary strategy can help to slow the progression of the disease. This is why it's so important for patients to be diagnosed with Lipedema as early as possible—even around puberty. There are a number of things patients can do at home or with the assistance of a licensed therapist, such as a certified lymphedema therapist (CLT), manual lymphatic drainage (MLD) therapist, Vodder therapist, certified lymphedema and wound therapist (CLWT), or a complete decongestive therapist (CDT).

Compression therapy falls into several categories:

Compression Garments

Virtually all patients with Lipedema will benefit from wearing compression garments. Patients who experience aggressive swelling need to be diligent in their use of higher-pressure garments. Patients with minimal swelling may find it beneficial to wear compression garments when they tend to swell—such as when traveling, at higher temperatures, or during exercise.

Compression garments are an important aspect of prevention, even for teenage patients. Patients who have significant swelling and leakiness should be almost living in compression garments. Stage 4 lipo-lymphedema patients should be using flat-knit garments that are commonly custom fitted. Compression garments may be covered by certain insurance plans, especially for advanced patients.

Bandaging

Advanced Lipedema patients, or those with lipo-lymphedema, may benefit from bandaging at certain times. This bandaging is typically performed by certified lymphatic therapists (CLT) who know how to bandage, or by patients at home who have learned how to bandage correctly at times when they are more congested.

FarrowWrap® garments are a range of adjustable compression devices that provide the same strong support as multilayered bandaging without the complexity of application. Available in a variety of styles, sizes, and compression classes, FarrowWraps help to reduce limb swelling and maintain volume reductions.

Manual Lymphatic Drainage Therapy

Manual lymphatic drainage (MLD) therapy is a specialized massage technique that helps promote the movement of lymphatic fluids from areas of swelling. It plays an important role in Lipedema and may be vital for certain patients.

Regular manual lymphatic drainage sessions with a qualified MLD therapist may help patients with rapidly progressing Lipedema, especially where they are starting to get more fibrosis. MLD therapy may be covered by certain insurance plans, but for patients who find an MLD therapist too cost-prohibitive, they can learn certain at-home tricks, available on the internet, that may be performed by themselves or by a significant other, family member, or friend.

Compression Pump Therapy

Compression pump therapy—such as the Flexitouch® system or Lymphopress Optimal Plus™—plays an important role in Lipedema treatment, particularly in advanced patients with prominent swelling. Compression pump therapy uses an air pump paired with a sleeve that fits over the affected extremity. Intermittent air pressure is applied to the sleeve, which in turn applies pressure to the extremity to redirect fluid to healthy regions of the body.

Compression pump therapy can be performed at home or in the office of a lymphatic therapist and may be covered by some insurance plans.

Fascia Blasters

A fascia blaster is a hard plastic tool, similar in appearance to a rod or stick, that can be used to massage areas of the body affected by Lipedema to improve circulation and promote lymphatic drainage.

Quadrivas Therapy

Quadrivas therapy, also known as manual subcutaneous adipose tissue therapy (SAT), is a type of deep tissue massage that was developed in Vietnam and adapted by Alyna Eekema of the Netherlands, who found great success using it to treat symptoms of Lipedema.

In the United States, Dr. Karen Herbst performed a pilot study of SAT therapy at the University of Arizona in 2016[ix] and found that in Lipedema patients, four weeks of SAT therapy improved tissue structure, leg function, and volume. All patients participating in the study felt SAT therapy was beneficial and would recommend it to other women with Lipedema. However, currently there are no practitioners of Quadrivas therapy in the United States.

OTHER THERAPIES

Vibrational Therapy

Whole-body vibrational therapy uses vibration at low frequencies to encourage lymphatic drainage and eliminate fluids and swelling from the body. Currently, there is no clinical proof that vibrational exercises improve Lipedema; however, many patients have found it to be very beneficial.

Aqua Therapy

Water exercises can be highly beneficial for Lipedema patients. The water supports the body by decreasing the effects of gravity, allowing for easier movement to strengthen muscles and to encourage the flow of lymph fluid and blood.

THE ROLE OF LIPOSUCTION IN LIPEDEMA

By the time Lipedema is diagnosed in many patients, they are in their thirties, forties, fifties, sixties, or seventies and have experienced years—or even decades—of the condition progressing with not only the gradual increase of Lipedema fat in the subcutaneous layer but also the effects of chronic inflammation which leads to fibrosis in the fat layer and increasing congestion.

Patients often become "maxed out" with trying different strategies to improve their symptoms and bodies. This is where the role of liposuction becomes an extremely important consideration. The patient may have already been on various respectful diets for years, as well as compression therapy, without any further improvement, or in some cases, worsening of their symptoms.

When Lipedema has progressed to this point, liposuction becomes the singular, most significant life-changing step a patient can take to treat their disease—and to prevent and manage its reoccurrence. Liposuction is not only important for the removal of the Lipedema fat but also for the decongestive benefits. A lot of the external treatments for Lipedema (such as compression therapy or manual lymphatic drainage) really can't compare with the benefits of internally removing that layer of fat and decongesting the fibrosis to create a healthier environment for the tissue and lymphatics. When performed correctly, liposuction will help to decongest entire areas of congestion, from the most proximal to the most distal.

The Two Main Goals of Lipedema Surgery:

1. Maximal disease treatment and prevention
2. Maximal cosmetic improvement

The role of liposuction should accomplish several goals in a patient with Lipedema:

Relieve Pain

Liposuction surgery will almost always greatly diminish or resolve the pain from Lipedema. Most patients can distinguish that their pain has resolved, oftentimes within hours or days of their surgery. They may have soreness from the liposuction itself, but they can distinguish that the soreness from surgery is very different from their Lipedema pain.

Reduce Swelling

Lipedema patients with swelling typically see significant improvements in their swelling after liposuction surgery. In my experience, patients fall into three categories.
For those in category one, the swelling essentially just goes away. As long as the patient is respectful of their dietary strategies after surgery, the swelling doesn't return to any significant degree.

Category two is the patient who still swells at certain times, possibly when they travel, exercise, or when in hot weather. This patient should still pay attention to that swelling, as it signifies that they may still need to wear compression garments at these times or continue with certain aspects of compression therapy.

Category three is the patient who has very aggressive swelling as part of their Lipedema. Typically, these patients will have prominent swelling prior to surgery. A small percentage of these patients are at significant risk of swelling reoccurring after surgery. These patients should continue consistent compression therapy after surgery, such as the regular use of compression garments or other compression modalities. In my experience, I would say this aggressive type of swelling occurs in less than 5 percent of patients with Lipedema.

A common question asked by a Lipedema patient is, "Will the

Lipedema come back after liposuction surgery?" In my extensive experience, it very rarely does. The small percentage of patients with aggressive swelling seem to be at the most risk of a reoccurrence of symptoms. In my practice, these patients are on strict, long-term compression therapy, even after surgery.

Resolve Misdiagnosed Symptoms

There are a number of misdiagnosed symptoms that I see greatly improve after liposuction surgery, such as plantar fasciitis. Patients may experience pain, tingling, or reduced sensation on the bottoms of their feet, and may possibly be misdiagnosed with peripheral neuropathy. I have treated many patients diagnosed with fibromyalgia who find their "fibromyalgia symptoms" have disappeared after surgery. This has also occurred with a condition called reflex sympathetic dystrophy that many Lipedema patients are diagnosed with by other doctors. Miraculously, after liposuction surgery, those symptoms typically resolve, which indicates that they were likely misdiagnoses. Those symptoms were primarily part of the patient's Lipedema symptoms and occurred because the fibrosis in the layer of fat was either affecting the peripheral nervous system or impeding lymphatic flow distally to those areas. Many patients signs and symptoms of Lipedema in their legs have been erroneously attributed to venous insufficiency. But by far the most common misdiagnosis is obesity, with its resulting treatment recommendations aimed at simply losing weight.

Improve Appearance

The role of liposuction surgery arguably is not only to treat the disease and its symptoms, but also to provide huge benefits in terms of the cosmetic improvements when liposuction is properly done.

Liposuction should achieve maximal functional improvement of the disease and the symptoms, reversal of progression, as well as maximum cosmetic improvements. In my practice, some advanced patients only care about the disease treatment and managing their symptoms. Stage 1 or 2 Lipedema patients who are not experiencing symptoms may primarily care about the way their legs look. But the benefit should be maximized in both areas—functional and cosmetic.

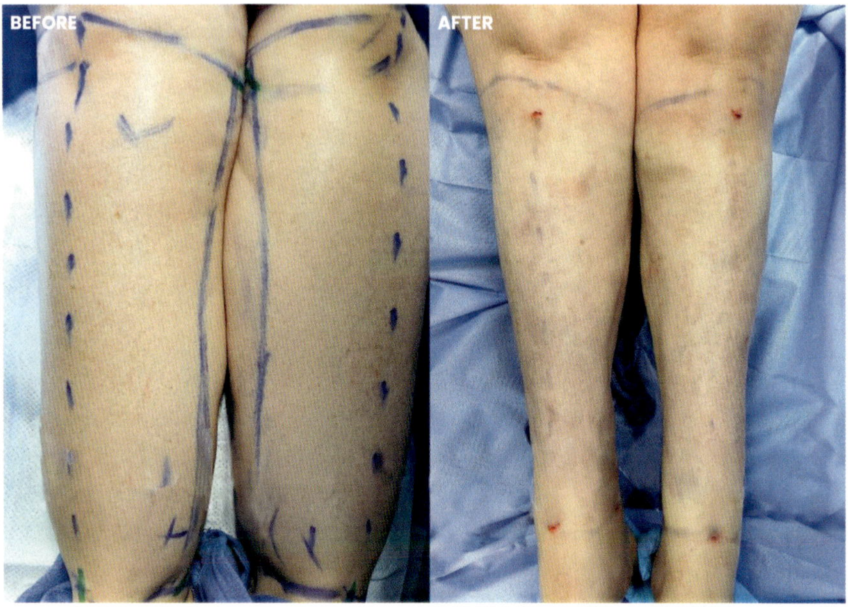

Above: Tangible cosmetic improvement can be seen in this patient's lower legs immediately post liposuction

WHY LIPEDEMA LIPOSUCTION DIFFERS FROM COSMETIC LIPOSUCTION

Liposuction for Lipedema is one of the most complicated and challenging forms of liposuction surgery. It requires extensive experience in liposuction of lipedema patients, a high technical proficiency, specific pre and post surgical protocols, and a dedicated surgical team of nurses and lymphatic therapists to provide the highest standards of care. Ideally the surgeon and center should be dedicated to Lipedema and not simply offering surgery for it.

The surgery is quite different from typical cosmetic liposuction for a number of reasons:

Lipedema Is a Disease

Treatment must be done with the disease in mind, rather than just focusing on the cosmetic improvements.

Complicated Areas

Lipedema affects complex parts of the body that most surgeons avoid, such as the calves, ankles, and forearms.

Circumferential Approach

Lipedema fat wraps around the entire body part, making it necessary to approach the unit circumferentially rather than as small, localized areas or strips.

Susceptible to Bruising

Since bruising is a prominent Lipedema symptom, it is important to proceed with the increased risk for bleeding and bruising in mind. This is one important reason why the proper preparation of the tissue by tumescent solution is so important.

Susceptible to DVT

Lipedema patients are at an increased risk for deep vein thrombosis

(DVT), requiring postsurgical anticoagulation.

Reduced Skin Elasticity

It is crucial to be mindful of the Lipedema patient's reduced skin elasticity due to coexisting Ehlers-Danlos syndrome.

Lymphatic Sparing

A lymphatic sparing approach is necessary for proper, safe Lipedema treatment.

Extensive Fibrosis

Removal of fibrosis and scar tissue is crucial for proper disease treatment.

PATTERNS OF FIBROSIS IN LIPEDEMA

Fibrosis is an important component of Lipedema and is a significant—if not the main—culprit of pain and possible damage leading to lipo-lymphedema. It is important for the Lipedema surgeon to understand its role in disease progression, the various types of fibrosis, and how to effectively deal with each type.

In my surgical experience with Lipedema patients, I have come to understand the different types of fibrosis and how they affect various symptoms and disease progression.

The four categories of fibrosis I have defined are:

1. **Nodular:** Typically cause pain or pressure.
2. **Weblike:** These patients tend to have softer "fluffy" fat and tend to be more prone to swelling.
3. **Dense:** These patients form a dense, almost concrete-like, fibrotic process. They tend to be the most prone to lymphatic damage, are slow to decongest, and are at higher risk for lipo-lymphedema.
4. **Granular:** Many patients primarily have a small, granular, sand-like fibrotic pattern, typically in the subdermal part of the superficial fat layer.

Each patient is unique in their fibrotic patterns. And many will have more than one type of fibrosis, although there exists a preponderance of generally one category. Some patients have numerous nodules while others have virtually none. Some patients have primarily a granular pattern with virtually no dense or weblike areas. Some patients quickly develop a dense pattern with no nodules.

The symptoms of the patient's disease is also dependent on the pattern of fibrosis. A stage 3 patient may have a weblike pattern with swelling and no pain, while a stage 1 patient may have a dense pattern with extreme pain. Interestingly, I have noticed that the type of pattern is almost always inherited as when I have treated sisters or a mother and daughter, they have typically shown the same fibrotic patterns.

PREOPERATIVE CONSIDERATIONS

There are a number of preoperative considerations in Lipedema patients that are important, and which differ from a cosmetic liposuction patient.

To begin with, every patient once diagnosed with Lipedema should be on a proper dietary strategy that is respectful for Lipedema. It is not only important for the prevention of further development, but even after surgery, patients should continue with the same respectful dietary strategy for Lipedema.

Compression therapy also plays an important role in virtually every patient's treatment for Lipedema. Swelling plays a role in this disease before—and many times after—surgery. Patients should get on the right type of compression strategy for themselves prior to surgery.

For patients with more advanced Lipedema (stages 3 or 4) or lipo-lymphedema, it is important for them to be on proper compression therapy prior to surgery. Many of the advanced patients I see have unhealthy fibrotic tissue and may have vascular compromise in their lower legs, causing the skin to turn darker colors or red. This compromised tissue needs to be in a much healthier place prior to proceeding with surgery. I recommend these patients be put on an aggressive presurgical compression protocol involving pump therapy or bandaging until it is safe to proceed with liposuction surgery.

In mild or moderate Lipedema patients (stages 1 or 2), it is not as imperative to be on a compression protocol prior to surgery, so I will typically proceed with surgery without having the patient undergo a strict presurgical protocol.

The lab work that most cosmetic liposuction patients complete prior to liposuction surgery should be expanded for Lipedema patients.

Many of these patients may have underlying hypercoagulable states, such as Factor V Leiden, that may need to be investigated. There may be an increased incidence of deep vein thrombosis (DVT) or clot formation, and some of the patients may already have a history of pulmonary emboli or anticoagulation therapy. It is important for the surgeon to coordinate with the patient's hematologist to design a perioperative protocol that may be more specific for avoiding complications of clot formation. In my practice, every patient is placed on Lovenox® anticoagulation therapy beginning the day after surgery for five days.

As with any surgery, the consultation is an important time to establish the preoperative considerations for each patient. In my practice, I define a very clear surgical treatment plan for every Lipedema patient, and I explain what the liposuction surgery is going to accomplish. This includes managing the patient's expectations in terms of the expected improvement of both physical symptoms and the cosmetic benefits of the surgery.

Cosmetically, if a patient has loose muscle or skin tone and liposuction is being performed for Lipedema, that patient should expect a certain degree of improvement with tightening depending on the elasticity and muscle tone of the area being treated.

If liposuction is performed well with proper respect for the skin, patients with good to excellent elasticity should see noticeable skin tightening. Patients with moderate loss of elasticity typically will benefit from a final step of skin tightening with Renuvion® or BodyTite®. Patients with poor elasticity should be considered for surgical tightening, such as with a brachioplasty or a thigh lift.

THE ANESTHETIC APPROACH TO LIPEDEMA

As outlined previously in this book, I strongly prefer to avoid liposuction under general anesthesia due to its negative impacts on safety, recovery, and results. I rarely use general anesthesia with liposuction. From an anesthetic standpoint, I either perform my surgeries under twilight sedation (MAC, or monitored anesthesia care) with an anesthesiologist or Certified Registered Nurse Anesthetist (CRNA), or purely under tumescent local anesthesia using mild sedation without an anesthesiologist.

For twilight sedation, the anesthesiologist is commonly going to use medications such as propofol, fentanyl, and midazolam—each of which should only be administered by a licensed anesthesiologist or a CRNA. In my practice, when I am performing surgery with an anesthesiologist, I am careful to not overly sedate the patient throughout the entire procedure, otherwise it's possible to begin to lose all the benefits of doing the surgery under tumescent, local anesthesia due to the lack of optimal patient positioning.

My strategy is to have the patient in a much deeper level of sedation while the first step is taking place—putting all the tumescent fluid into the tissue to prepare, numb, and hydrodissect. During infiltration of the tumescent fluid the patient may experience tolerable slight sensations of pinching. Then the sedation is lightened so the patient can assist by positioning themselves precisely throughout the surgery. The patient is able to tighten their muscles and assume certain positions, which becomes very important not only for the complete treatment of the disease but also for the maximum cosmetic improvement.

Various Anesthetic Approaches

- Tumescent local with mild sedation (no anesthesiologist or CRNA)
- Tumescent local plus MAC (monitored anesthesia care) or twilight sedation with an anesthesiologist or CRNA
- General anesthesia: intubation and gases with an anesthesiologist or CRNA

VARIOUS SURGICAL APPROACHES TO LIPEDEMA

Surgeons who specialize in Lipedema surgery typically approach it in one of three ways. One common approach is to debulk or spot treat specific areas where the Lipedema is more active, such as the medial knee area, the outer and inner thighs, or parts of the calves and ankles.

I call this debulking or spot treating because the patient will typically achieve an improvement of their symptoms by hitting those so-called hotspots of Lipedema. This approach may relieve a lot of the symptoms in those areas, but it really isn't the most ideal way of approaching Lipedema because the process of the disease is occurring in the entire area circumferentially. By just approaching from a spot-treatment standpoint, it's not a complete surgery because areas of Lipedema are left behind that could become more active and problematic. And certainly, from a cosmetic standpoint, it's not really the best approach to create the right type of three-dimensional shape to the entire "cosmetic unit".

In my experience, this approach is often performed by surgeons who are not aware the patient has been diagnosed with Lipedema, or they may even be unaware of Lipedema itself as a condition, and so they spot treats areas for improvement, only to have the patient return years later with worsening symptoms in other areas. This is a large category of the revision liposuction surgery I perform, where I will go back in and balance the whole "cosmetic unit" properly and completely.

The next common approach is what I call the strip approach. In this approach, either the outer or inner parts of the legs, or alternately the anterior half of the legs, are treated with one surgery. Then, in another surgery, the posterior parts of the legs are treated. I call this the strip approach because you're doing strips of the leg and generally connecting them later on.

In my practice, I reserve the strip approach for about 2 to 3 percent of my patients who have very advanced Lipedema or lipo-lymphedema where I do not want to use the circumferential approach—mainly because these patients are very advanced, and their tissue is starting to become unhealthy with fibrosis, congestion, or lymphatic damage. There is typically too much congestion in their tissue, and the circumferential approach will generally prolong their recovery.

When performing liposuction on these advanced patients, I typically start with a semi-circumferential strip of the medial parts of the legs all the way down to the feet, or I start with the lateral part of the leg and then move around the leg in strips to connect those two areas in a semi-circumferential process or pattern in two surgeries.

The final way of approaching Lipedema is with a technique I developed approximately twenty-five years ago, which I call the circumferential 360° approach for Lipedema. It is similar in technique to the circumferential approach for cosmetic liposuction patients, where I am treating the entire "cosmetic unit" circumferentially at one time. This is the technique I use for over 95 percent of my Lipedema patients.

I find the circumferential approach is much better for the Lipedema patients who are candidates for it, because from a disease treatment standpoint, Lipedema is a circumferential disease, and it can be treated all the way around in one surgery. From a cosmetic standpoint, I find it far superior because it gives me the ability to completely blend everything at one time and not have to connect areas at separate times. For example, when I treat the thigh area, it is done from the knee all the way up to the groin area circumferentially. The calf and ankle areas are treated from the knee down to the ankle completely circumferentially.

If I treat the torso of a Lipedema patient, it is done circumferentially, as are the arms. If a patient notices their arms are full, they begin to understand that it's not just the back parts of the arms, like in cosmetic patients, but the entire upper arm area (and many times, the forearms) that need to be treated, so it is blended the whole way around. There is great benefit to being able to blend everything at one time for optimal cosmetic results. However, this approach is far more technically challenging for many reasons.

Various Surgical Approaches to Lipedema

- Spot treat/debulk
- Strip (medial/lateral or anterior/posterior)
- Complete circumferential 360°

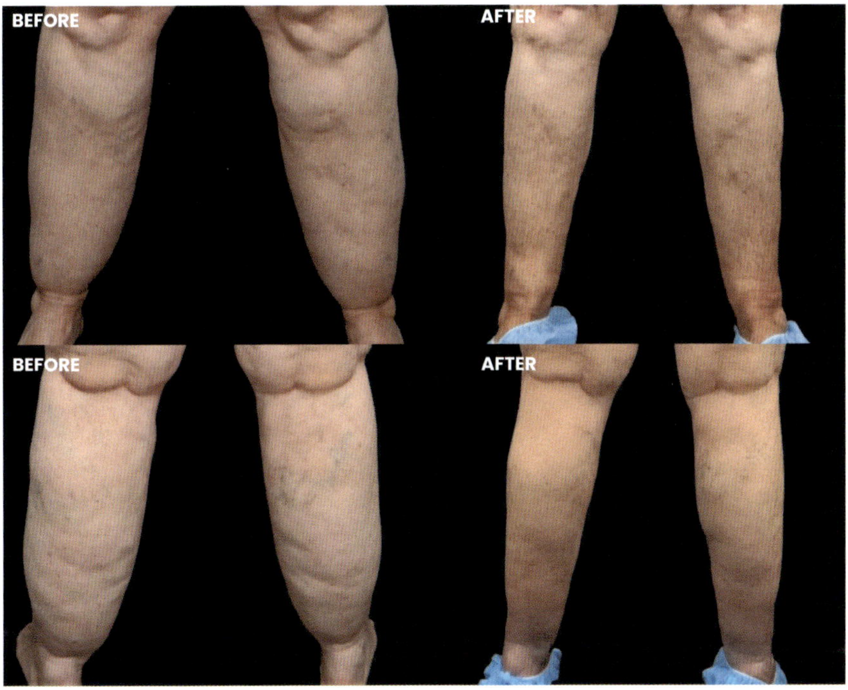

Above: This stage 3 Lipedema patient received circumferential liposuction to their lower legs

THE TOOLS FOR LIPEDEMA LIPOSUCTION SURGERY

The tools used for Lipedema liposuction surgery are similar to those used for cosmetic liposuction surgery, as outlined in Section 1: Cosmetic Liposuction. As with cosmetic liposuction, it is important for the patient to trust in the skills of their surgeon and not only in the tools being used. The surgeon should be examining the patient's body for overall "balance and proportion" with an understanding of "cosmetic units", and they should be respectful of the skin. These factors are by far more important than the tools that are being used.

In my practice, I have progressively and carefully incorporated devices over the years that I feel enhance my already defined technique with liposuction surgery. With Lipedema, I have found that each tool has a very specific role when I am performing surgery.

Some tools are very good at mechanically releasing the tissue, while others (such as VASER) have a role in the emulsification of the fat layer and further release of fibrotic tissue. I find power-assisted liposuction helpful for the mechanical release of the fibrous tissue, especially with the suction turned off.

Water-assisted liposuction is good for putting in the tumescent fluid and for the proper preparation of the tissue, but it is not as ideal for releasing the fibrosis and scar tissue associated with Lipedema.

I use laser in a specific way for very fibrotic nodules of Lipedema, or sometimes in patients with Dercum disease due to its focused high peak temperature. Skin tightening is a final step in certain patients. I use either Renuvion® or BodyTite® for maximal tightening in patients with moderate loss of elasticity.

Functional and Cosmetic Benefit by Tool

	Fibrosis Release	Emulsification	Skin Tightening	Cellulite	Nodules/Dercums
WAL	★★	★	★	★	★
Vaser	★★★★	★★★★★	★★	★★★★	★
PAL	★★★★★	★★★	★	★★	★★
Laser	★★	★★	★★★	★★	★★★★
Radiofrequency	★	★★	★★★★★	★	★★
Renuvion	★★	★★★	★★★★★	★★★	★★

THE PROCESS OF LIPOSUCTION FOR LIPEDEMA PATIENTS

The process of liposuction for Lipedema patients is a multistep process, similar to my process for cosmetic liposuction patients.

Step 1: Tumescent Anesthesia

Using water-assisted liposuction, I prepare the tissue with tumescent anesthesia by infiltrating a dilute lidocaine solution of local anesthetic combined with epinephrine and sodium bicarbonate into the tissue until it becomes firm (tumescent) and white in color. The fluids from the tumescent anesthesia hydrodissects the treatment field, helping to release and break apart the subcutaneous layer, preparing it for the next step. The complete tumescence of the subcutaneous layer is an important preparatory step and should be differentiated from incomplete tumescence, such as the wet technique. If done properly, it also reduces bleeding and bruising. Water-assisted liposuction (WAL) is more of a layperson term; the correct medical terminology is tumescent anesthesia. If done properly, there is only slight tolerable discomfort with a sensation of mild pinching.

Step 2: Debulk and Mechanical Release

The second step is the removal of the deeper layer of fat. This is an important step for Lipedema patients. It is round one of liposculpture, and it is done to sculpt the layer down to 20 percent or less and to further break open the scar tissue. Using power-assisted liposuction, the vibration works to not only debulk and remove the fat but also to mechanically release the fibrous tissue.

Step 3: Emulsification with VASER

The ultrasonic energy with VASER is an excellent tool to melt and emulsify the fat. This step also further releases the fibrosis, especially the micro and smaller fibrosis under the skin, melting and releasing it. VASER is excellent for improving the appearance of cellulite in both Lipedema and cosmetic patients because it transects and releases the fibrous bands that cause the rippled appearance.

Step 4: Fine Sculpting

My fourth step is fine sculpting using smaller cannulas to perform precise sculpting of the tissue as the layer gets thinner. This step has to be done with great respect for the skin to achieve the best results cosmetically, because the layer of fat has already been brought down by step two. In this step it is important for the patient to tighten their muscles to create a firm platform, and for the surgeon and technician to be stretching and supporting the skin in a uniform manner. When properly done, this step assists in the even contraction of the skin without causing ripples.

Step 5: Skin Tightening

I employ skin tightening in about 50 percent of my patients using either Renuvion® or BodyTite®. Renuvion is an ionized helium gas that rapidly heats the skin and tissue. I like to use Renuvion in larger areas, such as the torso or thighs, for its ability to contract the skin in a uniform fashion. I use BodyTite, which is a radio-frequency device for areas such as the knee or the "banana roll" underneath the buttocks.

If patients have excellent elasticity of their skin tissue, they generally do not need this step. In certain areas of the body where the skin is taut, such as on the calves and ankles, I rarely use this additional tightening step.

Patients with an extreme loss of elasticity or thin, wrinkling skin will likely benefit more from a surgical tightening procedure than from this step.

Renuvion or BodyTite is typically used in areas of moderate loss of elasticity such as on the thighs, arms, or abdomen, where a patient wants to avoid a surgical tightening procedure such as a brachioplasty, thigh lift, or abdominoplasty.

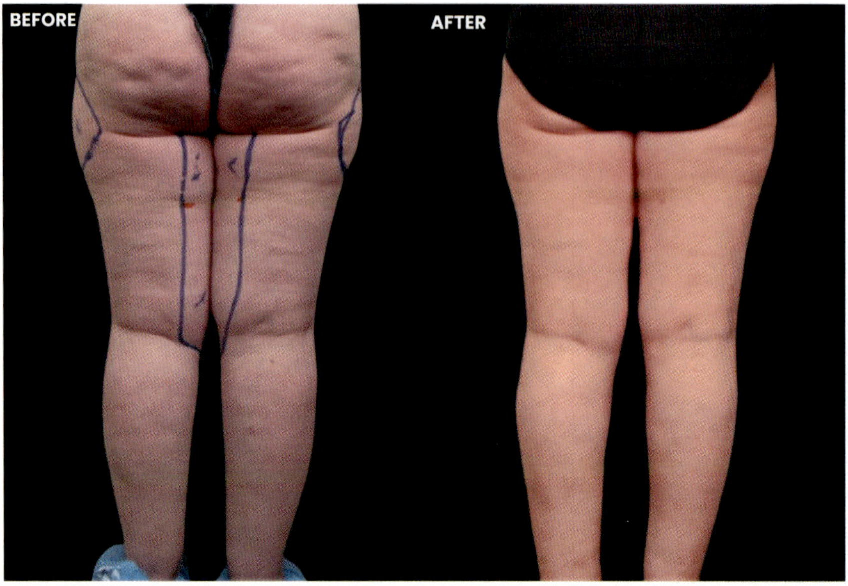

Above: This stage 1 Lipedema patient received liposuction to their upper and lower legs

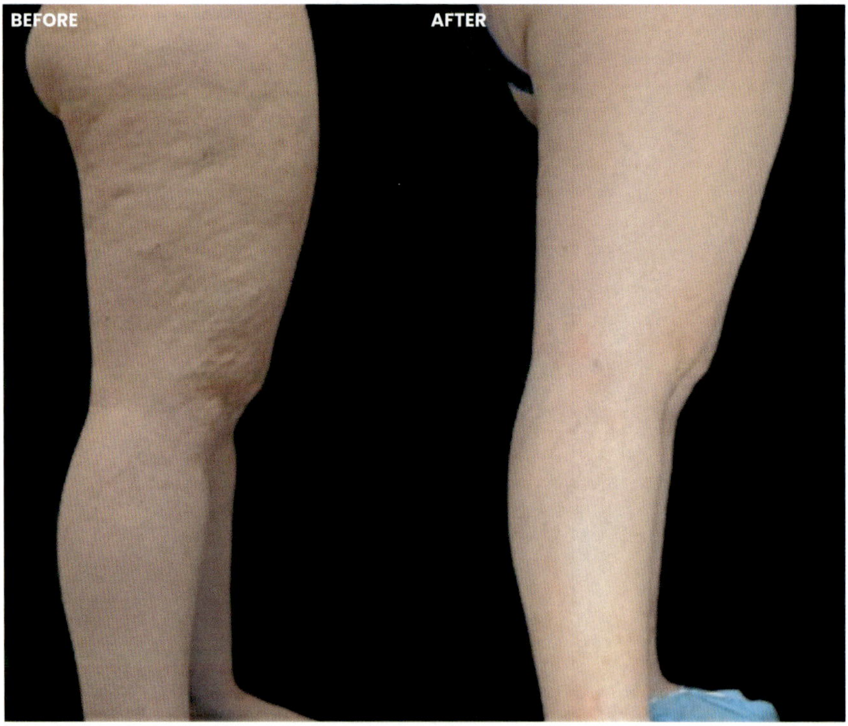

Above: Visible textural improvement can be seen on this stage 1 Lipedema patients' thighs after liposuction

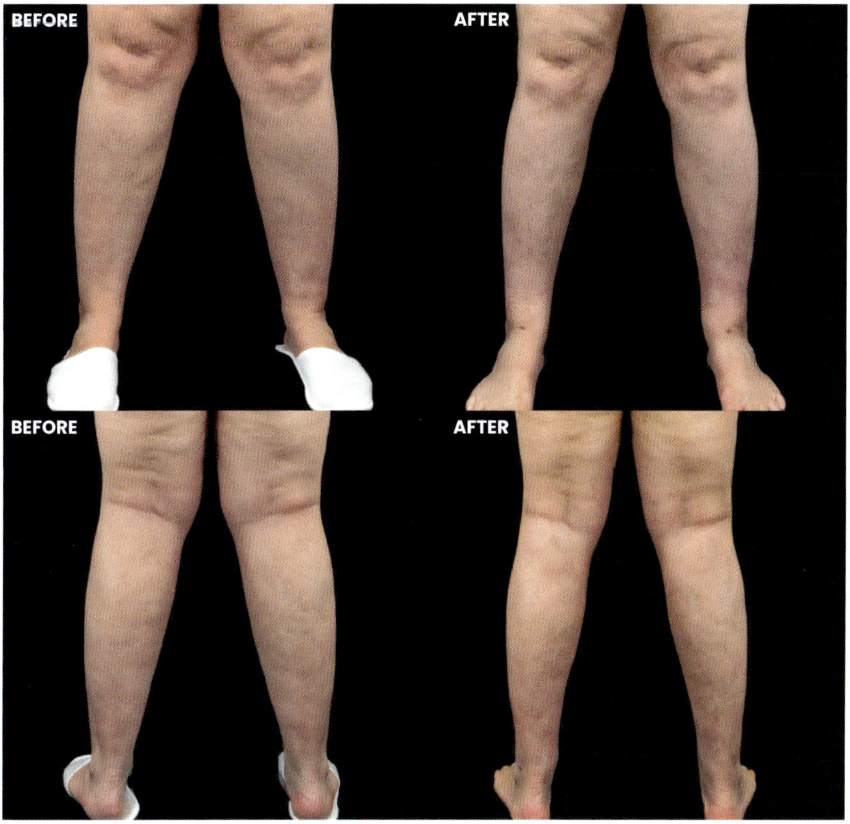

Above: This stage 2 Lipedema patient received circumferential 360° liposuction to their calves, ankles, and thighs.

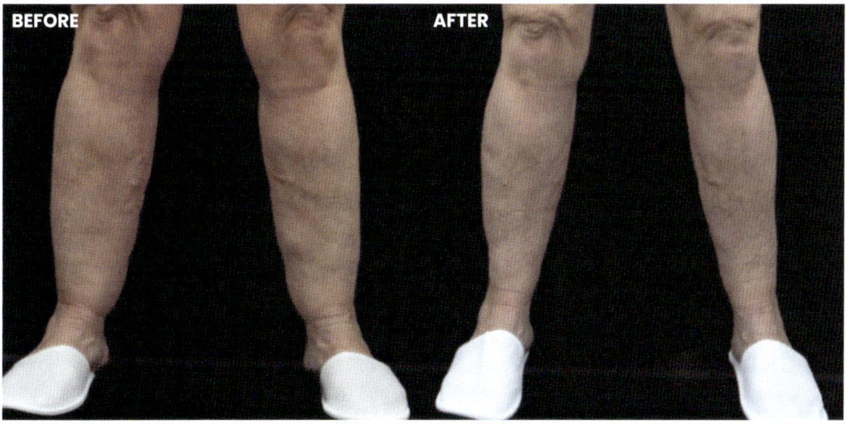

Above: Circumferential 360° liposuction was performed on the calves and ankles of this stage 2 Lipedema patient.

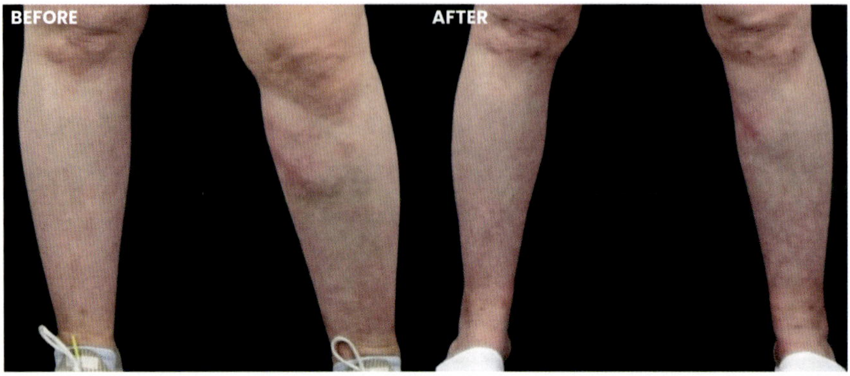

Above: This stage 2 Lipedema patient received circumferential liposuction to their lower legs

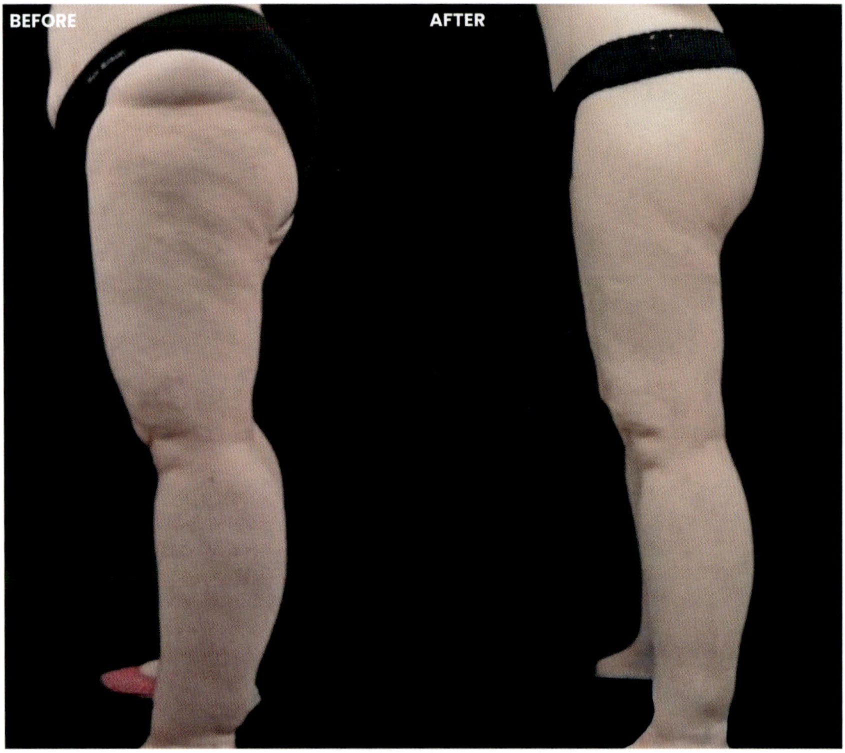

Above: Liposuction was performed on the full legs, hips, and abdomen of this stage 2 Lipedema patient

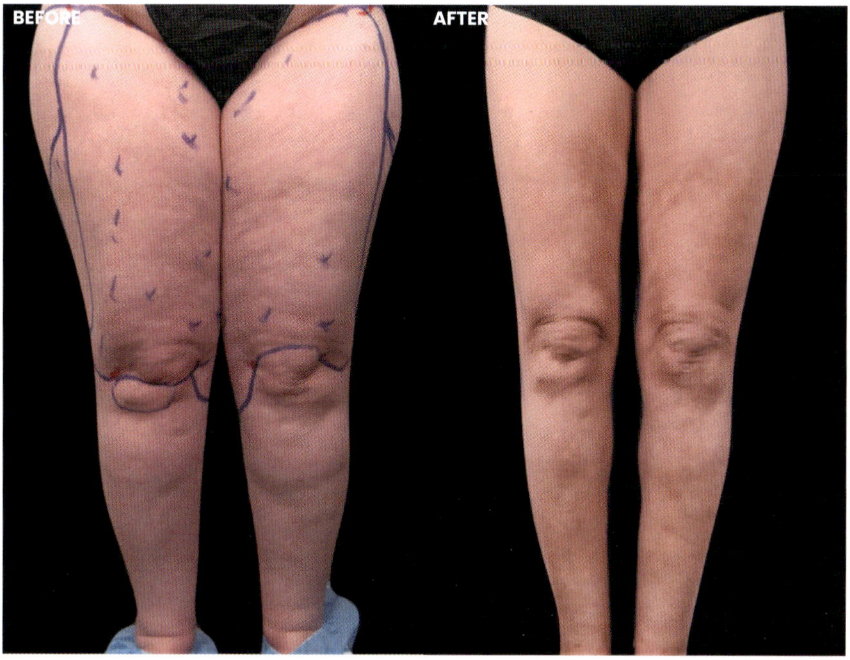

Above: Tangible cosmetic improvement can be seen in in the upper and lower legs of this stage 2 Lipedema patient after liposuction

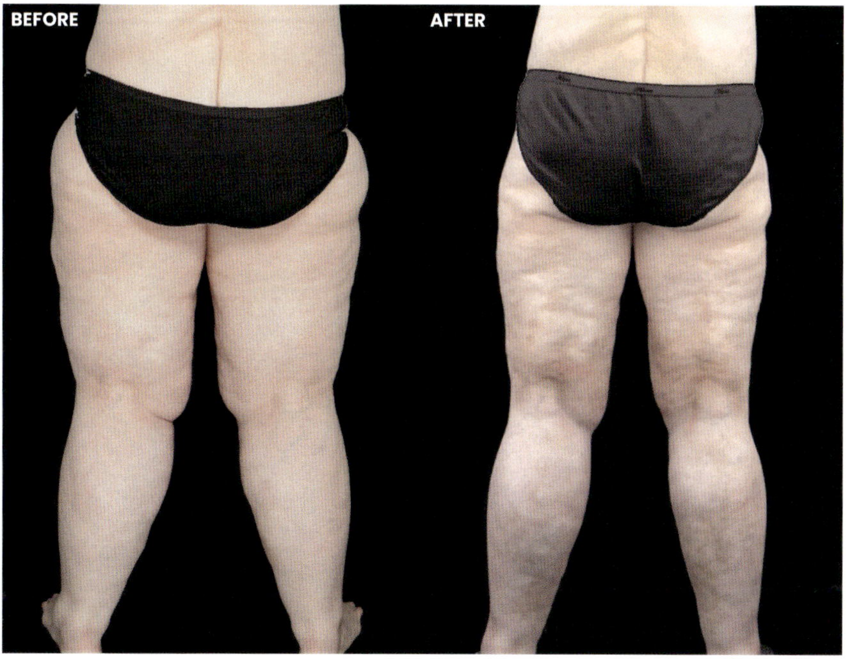

Above: This stage 3 Lipedema patient received circumferential 360° liposuction to their calves, ankles and thighs.

SURGICAL TIGHTENING

Many Lipedema patients have a moderate to advanced loss of skin elasticity. This often presents itself in the upper arms, inner thigh area, and torso. These patients may need to consider a surgical tightening procedure in addition to liposuction if the loss of elasticity is advanced.

Patients with a mild or moderate loss of skin elasticity can have improvement and tightening without cutting the skin, using either Renuvion® or BodyTite®. If the loss of elasticity has become more advanced, I discuss the consideration of a surgical tightening procedure for these patients. If the patient is open to this, they consult with my plastic surgeon.

One of the most common areas where this occurs is on the upper arm. An arm lift—also known as a brachioplasty—can often be performed concomitantly with liposuction surgery. If the patient is more advanced, it may be considered as a secondary surgical

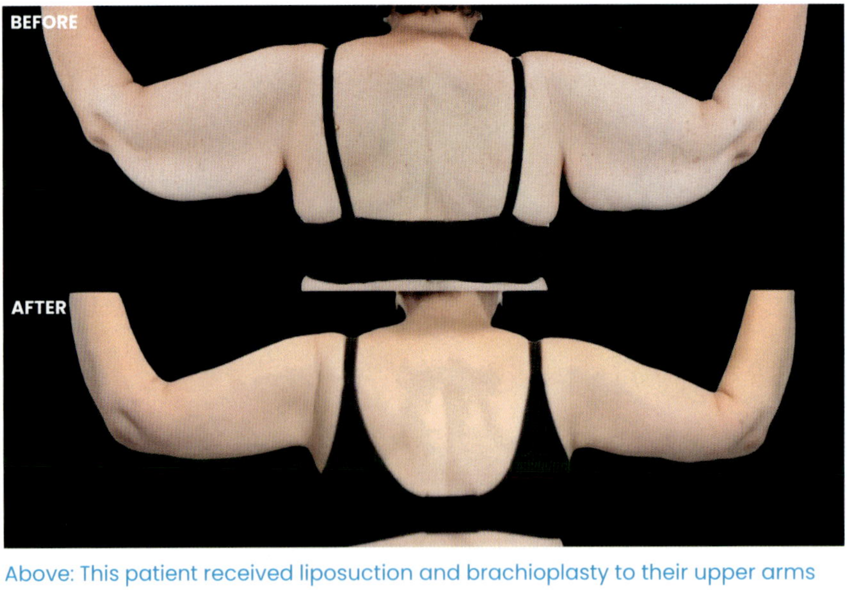

Above: This patient received liposuction and brachioplasty to their upper arms

tightening procedure after liposuction surgery. The brachioplasty involves the removal of excess skin and will typically result in a thin surgical scar on the inner part of the arm. Brachioplasty can sometimes be done at the same time as liposuction, but it may be done separately in more advanced patients to achieve a better cosmetic result and reduce recovery issues.

The thighs are the next area of consideration for surgical tightening. A thigh lift, or thighplasty, procedure is generally a longer and more complicated procedure than a brachioplasty. I reserve this procedure for my Lipedema patients who have a more advanced loss of elasticity of their thigh skin. For patients with mild to moderate loss of elasticity, typically Renuvion or BodyTite will give quite a good degree of tightening to avoid surgical tightening and can also tighten other areas of the entire thigh unit that a thigh lift would not address.

In some patients a thigh lift can be performed concomitantly with liposuction surgery, but in my experience, it may be better and safer to do it as a separate procedure weeks or months after liposuction surgery has been performed. Thigh-lift procedures are typically performed with an incision and scar in the inguinal crease of the thigh but may also involve a vertical scar that goes down a certain degree of the upper inner thigh skin.

The third area where surgical tightening procedures are considered in Lipedema patients is the torso, with a potential tummy tuck procedure (abdominoplasty). Commonly patients with Lipedema who have put on a lot of weight may have a lot of skin laxity. I often perform liposuction on their torso partially for cosmetic reasons, but sometimes Lipedema is also involved in their abdomen. The consideration of a tummy tuck will arise similarly to other areas. If the loss of elasticity is not too significant, Renuvion or BodyTite will typically tighten the area well, but for more advanced skin laxity, a tummy tuck should be considered.

In my practice, a tummy tuck or abdominoplasty is typically performed weeks or months after circumferential liposuction of the torso. This is done in a staged manner to not only reduce complications but to also release all of the fibrotic tissue and prepare the area for the abdominoplasty. This staged approach in Lipedema patients will reduce complications and achieve a better cosmetic result.

A tummy tuck can be performed as a mini tummy tuck or as a full tummy tuck. The belly button is typically removed and repositioned as part of this surgery.

Categories of Skin Elasticity

Good to excellent: Typically no additional skin-tightening step necessary

Moderate: Typically good candidate for additional skin-tightening step with Renuvion or Bodytite

Poor: Typically considered for surgical excision of redundant skin with either arm or thigh lift

LIPEDEMA, VARICOSE VEINS, AND VENOUS INSUFFICIENCY

Varicose veins and venous insufficiency are a common issue for many women, and they often become more pronounced with age. They are the result of weakened or damaged valves that cause increased pressure and dilation of the veins. Lipedema also tends to exacerbate varicose veins. Many Lipedema patients have had their veins treated prior to having Lipedema liposuction surgery and have found treatments such as sclerotherapy or endovenous laser ablation to be unsuccessful.

In my experience with Lipedema patients who have varicose veins or venous insufficiency, it is almost always better to treat the Lipedema first with properly done liposuction surgery. The reason for this is that the release of fibrosis and decongestion from liposuction greatly reduces the hydrostatic pressure in the tissues surrounding the veins and reduces pressure in the veins. This tends to improve the varicose veins and venous insufficiency, but more importantly, it allows for more successful subsequent venous therapy, if needed. This is one more reason why proper tumescent anesthesia with fluid should always be given as a preparatory step to cause vasoconstriction and reduce bleeding during Lipedema liposuction surgery.

ORTHOPEDIC SURGERY AND LIPEDEMA

Approximately one-third of the patients I see for consultation prior to surgery have either had orthopedic knee surgery or have knee issues that need to be addressed by an orthopedist. The bulk of congestion, swelling, and fibrosis, along with being overweight contributes to ongoing stress on the knee joints. Medial knee fullness from the Lipedema also creates stress on the knees as the more advanced patients may not be able to bring their knees close enough together as they ambulate.

This underscores the importance of prevention and proper treatment of Lipedema before unfortunate knee damage requires surgery. Insurance companies should recognize this as one more reason to provide coverage for the treatment of Lipedema.

To make things further complicated, most orthopedic surgeons will not operate on a patient with a high BMI index and expect them to lose weight first (which may be all but impossible for advanced patients) or even recommend bariatric surgery.

In these advanced patients, my strategy is to proceed with the Lipedema surgery first. This decongests the area around the knees and reduces the weight and stress on the knee joints. Ultimately this makes the orthopedic surgeon happy in that the patient and the surgical area they may operate on are healthier, leading to a safer and less complicated recovery.

POSTOPERATIVE RECOVERY FOR LIPEDEMA PATIENTS

Lipedema is a disease, and although the postoperative recovery is similar to that of cosmetic liposuction, there are important specific considerations, especially with regard to compression.

Lipedema patients, unlike cosmetic patients, have an increased risk of clot formation due to scar tissue and congestion. Many of these patients have hypercoagulable states and decreased mobility after surgery. In my practice, I place every patient on a postoperative prophylactic anticoagulation regimen with Lovenox®, starting the day after each surgery and continuing for five days.

Patients with more significant risks of clot formation, such as those with a history of deep vein thrombosis (DVT) or pulmonary emboli, should have their postoperative anticoagulation care coordinated by both the surgeon and their hematologist. If patients were on anticoagulation therapy prior to surgery, they typically will stop for twenty-four to forty-eight hours and resume a day or two after surgery is performed.

As with my cosmetic patients, the majority of patients will return to where they are staying and will remain under the care of a responsible companion throughout the evening of the surgery. Sometimes, members of my support staff will spend the evening with the patient. If the patient is older or has significant medical issues, it may be recommended that a nurse spend the evening with them, or that they stay at an aftercare facility for the evening of the surgery.

Patients are provided instructions on how to look after the areas. There is typically draining and oozing of a blood-tinged clear to pinkish solution during the twenty-four to thirty-six hours after surgery. Patients are instructed to wear pads to absorb the leakage. I have never had the need to place surgical drains. Immediately after surgery, patients are placed into surgical compression garments, which they will wear twenty-four hours a day for one month, after which they are reassessed, and if decongesting in a linear fashion, they can reduce to wearing the compression garments for twelve hours a day for another month.

Patients are advised to resume a normal diet immediately after surgery and are instructed to hydrate well by drinking a glass of water every hour for eight to twelve hours. Intravenous fluids may also be given in the recovery room, and some patients receive IV hydration the following day.

The day after surgery, the patient returns to my clinic for a postoperative check. The compression garment is removed, and the areas are evaluated in terms of proper recovery. If the incision points have stopped oozing, a bandage will be applied with antibiotic ointment to each incision for several days until they completely close. The patient will begin a postop compression therapy regimen of manual lymphatic drainage twice a week for several weeks after the surgery. Lovenox anticoagulation is begun the day after surgery and is continued for five days to prevent any clot (DVT) formation.

For out-of-town patients, manual lymphatic drainage therapy is performed daily for three days postoperatively. Advanced Stage 3 or 4 patients are typically bandaged and wrapped during this period. Most patients are ready to fly home three days after surgery. On the flight home they are instructed to get up and walk around for a few minutes every two hours. By the time they return home, most patients are able to resume most of their routine daily activities.

For the first four days after surgery, the patient will shower in their compression garment. Lipedema patients may feel lightheaded when the pressure of the garment is released after surgery because they have fluid shifts and are prone to postural hypotension. Showering in the garment helps reduce dizziness.

When the garment is removed after the first four days, a moderate amount of bruising is to be expected. Lipedema patients are prone to bruising, which manifests itself even after surgery, and unlike my cosmetic patients, they will have a moderate degree of bruising for two to three weeks post surgery.

If decongestion is going well after that first month, the patient will switch over to wearing their compression garment for twelve hours a day for the second month post surgery.

Depending on how they are feeling on the day after surgery, I encourage my patients to resume light activity, such as going for short walks, which they will gradually increase each day. Patients who are feeling tired, weak, or uncomfortable are encouraged to take very short walks with a companion by their side. Intense exercise should be avoided for approximately three to four weeks after the surgery.

Patients start to see improvements in the first month after surgery. Most of their symptoms have already greatly improved or gone away. From a cosmetic standpoint, patients see improvements for up to twelve months post surgery, particularly if additional skin-tightening procedures such as Renuvion® have been performed, which can take up to eighteen months for the final tightening to take place.

Swelling in Lipedema patients can be slower to resolve compared to cosmetic patients, and this is especially true in patients with more congestion. The majority of patients tend to decongest in a linear fashion, but there is a small percentage of patients who, in the short-term, become more congested during the first few weeks or months after surgery. I call these patients "delayed decongesters."

In my experience, you can't always predict which patients may become more congested early on. One would think that this may be most common in more advanced patients, which is generally the case, especially if they have lipo-lymphedema. But sometimes, even stage 1 or 2 Lipedema patients will become more congested in the short-term and will have delayed lymphatic decongestion.

These patients will need more aggressive postoperative decongestion therapy. Some may need to be bandaged from very early on, and for several days up to two weeks. Some may benefit from compression pump therapy in the postoperative recovery process. But overall, the vast majority of patients decongest in a linear fashion and see great improvements in their swelling long-term.

THE LONG-TERM PREVENTION OF LIPEDEMA

The long-term prevention of Lipedema is an important topic. When discussing treatment options for this disease, patients will commonly ask if their Lipedema will come back after surgery, and if so, why it might come back.

And again, we don't completely understand Lipedema. But we do know a lot about it, and we're beginning to learn more. Lipedema is not only a process of fat overgrowth; there is also an involvement of inflammation and fibrosis, and the leakiness in the lymphatic system of the body.

Patients often ask me if their Lipedema will come back. I can only speak from my extensive experience treating Lipedema patients for many years. It very rarely comes back to any significant degree after liposuction surgery, and I've been following many of my patients for over twenty years.

After liposuction surgery, it is extremely important for patients to pay attention to their dietary strategies so they can prevent the reoccurrence of Lipedema. Similar to when younger pubescent patients are diagnosed with Lipedema, using preventative strategies, such as following a respectful Lipedema diet, can effectively slow or halt disease progression.

When I see patients who are in their thirties, forties, fifties, or sixties, and liposuction surgery is required, the process of decongesting the area, removing the fat, and releasing the fibrosis ultimately gives that compromised tissue a clean, fresh start, almost like taking them back to how their bodies may have been prior to the onset of Lipedema. From that point on, it becomes important for them to pay attention to doing everything they can to not have their symptoms return.

Regarding hormonal balance, patients will often ask if they should have surgery prior to a pregnancy or menopause. In my experience, if liposuction is performed prior to any hormonal changes, it is helpful in preventing a flare of symptoms when hormonal changes are present. I have had numerous patients who have become pregnant within a year after their surgeries without experiencing a flare of their Lipedema.

After liposuction surgery, patients should still pay attention to swelling. There are typically three types of patients in regard to long-term postoperative swelling.

The first type of patient doesn't tend to swell anymore and may not need compression garments or decongestive therapy.

The second type of patient may swell at certain times and should pay attention to what triggers may bring on the swelling, such as when they exercise, when it is hot, or during air travel or longer car travel. Even years after liposuction surgery, this swelling likely signifies that the patient should wear compression garments or may need compression therapy at those times.

The third type of patient unfortunately continues to experience swelling after surgery. In my experience, this occurs in less than 1 percent of patients, and they are at the greatest risk of their Lipedema symptoms reoccurring. These patient typically have very aggressive Lipedema with profound swelling prior to surgery. Many of them have aggressive lipo-lymphedema. These patients will still need to do aggressive compression therapy, such as wearing compression garments, or undergoing MLD or pump therapy as part of a lifelong treatment strategy.

We don't completely know why Lipedema doesn't return after liposuction surgery. But removing the fat and decongesting the area with liposuction, the contraction of the tissue should greatly reduce the chance of leakiness of the lymphatics and the development of fat in the future.

For some patients, years down the line, it may be a consideration to go back in and try to make further improvements. In my experience, in the thousands of patients I have treated over many years, it is rare that a patient that has been treated properly with liposuction surgery would need to go back for repeat procedures.

ABOUT THE AUTHOR

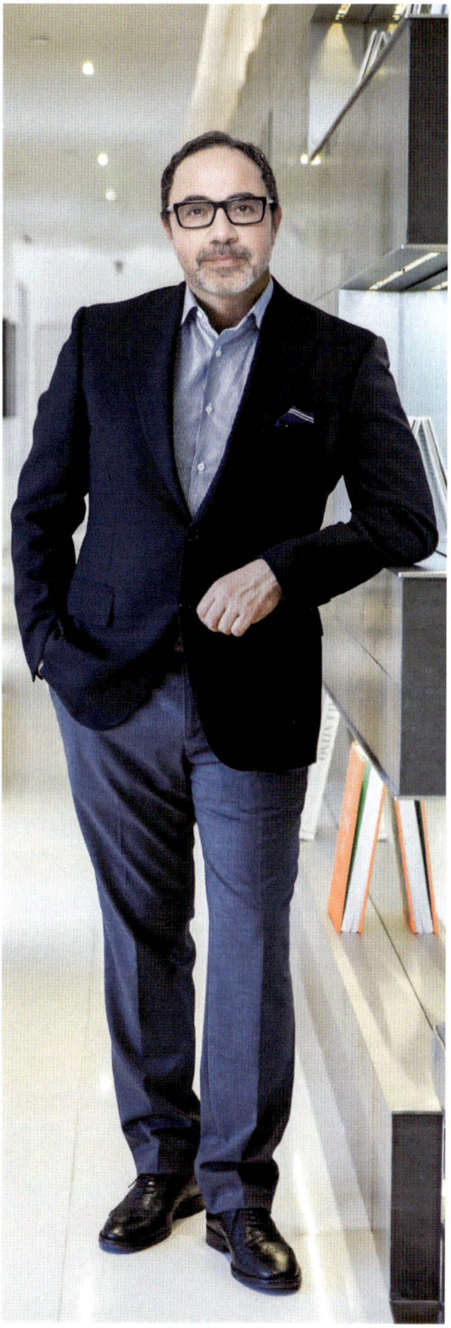

Dr. David Amron is the founder and medical director of The Roxbury Institute®, with locations in Beverly Hills, California, and Salt Lake City, Utah. Dr. Amron has devoted the past thirty years of his professional career to mastering and advancing the art and philosophy of a singular procedure: liposculpture surgery. He has honed and perfected his skills in over twelve thousand liposuction surgeries in the highly competitive world of Beverly Hills, where much of his practice is made up of patients from around the world seeking his expertise—whether it be for his Natural Def Lipo technique, his expertise in complicated revision work, or to transform the life of a patient suffering from Lipedema.

In the world of body sculpting, Dr. Amron has designed a revolutionary philosophy based on sound principles and advanced techniques. In this book he outlines his unique, essential concepts of "balance and proportion", the "cosmetic unit", the "safe plane", the five-step approach, and many others as part of his structured, systematic approach to body contouring.

As the pioneer of Lipedema surgery in the United States, Dr. Amron has trained surgeons from around the world in his advanced approach to liposuction for the treatment of Lipedema. He has established the Advanced Lipedema Treatment (ALT) program within the Roxbury Institute, as well as the Lipedema Society™ which is aimed at increasing awareness of this ignored disease among patients and health-care professionals. In addition, he recently released an educational online series entitled Lippy Logic™.

A believer in educating his peers and forwarding his field, Dr. Amron is widely published in medical journal articles and textbooks on dermatologic surgery. He is passionate about lecturing and teaching his unique techniques and philosophies for liposuction and Lipedema surgery, both nationally and abroad.

As a key opinion leader, Dr. Amron has been featured extensively in the media, including in print, on television, and on radio. He has contributed to numerous print articles such as the Wall Street Journal and Los Angeles Times. Dr. Amron has appeared on countless television networks and shows, including BBC, The Learning Channel (TLC), the TODAY show, and 60 Minutes Australia, and as a cast member of the Netflix series, Celebrity Plastic Surgeons of Beverly Hills.

Additionally, for a period of two years, Dr. Amron hosted the popular Los Angeles-based radio show, A Cut Above, which focused on educating the public on the do's and don'ts of cosmetic surgery and the avoidance of falling prey to deceitful marketing tactics.

Dr. Amron is a fellow of multiple prestigious medical and surgical societies including the American Academy of Cosmetic Surgery and the American Society for Dermatologic Surgery.

This book provides invaluable insights for any patient considering liposuction surgery, as well as pearls of wisdom for surgeons looking to advance their approaches or techniques for this procedure.

Outside of medicine, Dr. Amron is an accomplished guitarist, singer, and songwriter. He enjoys horseback riding, fast cars, and skiing. Dr. Amron resides in Beverly Hills, California, with his wife and four children.

NOTES

i American Society of Plastic Surgeons, *Plastic Surgery Statistics Report 2010*, https://www.plasticsurgery.org/documents/News/Statistics/2010/plastic-surgery-statistics-full-report-2010.pdf.

ii American Society of Plastic Surgeons, *Plastic Surgery Statistics Report 2019*, https://www.plasticsurgery.org/documents/News/Statistics/2019/plastic-surgery-statistics-full-report-2019.pdf.

iii Grazer, F. M., and, R. H. de Jong RH,. "Fatal Outcomes from Liposuction: Census Survey of Cosmetic Surgeons,." *Plastic and Reconstructive Surgery*. 2000 Jan;105(1), 436–448. https://doi.org/10.1097/00006534-200001000-00070

iv Torp, K.D., Metheny E., and Simon L. V., *Lidocaine Toxicity* (Treasure Island, Florida: StatPearls Publishing, 2020), https://www.ncbi.nlm.nih.gov/books/NBK482479/tics-full-report-2019.pdf.

v Torp, K.D., Metheny E., and Simon L. V., *Lidocaine Toxicity* (Treasure Island, Florida: StatPearls Publishing, 2020), https://www.ncbi.nlm.nih.gov/books/NBK482479/tics-full-report-2019.pdf.

vi Allen, E. V., and E. A. Hines, " EA. Lipedema of the Legs: A Syndrome Characterized by Fat Legs and Orthostatic Eedema,". *Mayo Clinic Proceedings* 15 (March. 1940) March;15: 184–187.

vii Wold, L., E. A. Hines, and E. V. Allen, "Lipedema of the Legs: A Syndrome Characterized by Fat Legs and Edema," *Annals of Internal Medicine* 34 (1951): 1243–50, https://doi.org/10.7326/0003-4819-34-5-1243.

viii Ehrlich, C., E. Iker, and K. L. Herbst, *Lymphedema and Lipedema Nutrition Guide* (Lymph Notes, 2016).

ix Herbst, K. L., C. Ussery, and A. Eekema, "Pilot Study: Whole Body Manual Subcutaneous Adipose Tissue (SAT) Therapy Improved Pain and SAT Structure in Women with Lipedema," *Hormone Molecular Biology and Clinical Investigation* 33, no. 2 (September 2017), https://doi.org/10.1515/hmbci-2017-0035.